Freestyle 2018

The Ultimate Weight Loss Program for a New You

By Abby Muller

TABLE OF CONTENTS

INSTANT POT PASTA & GRAIN DISHES. 118

SOUPS, STEWS, CHILIES 125

INSTANT POT DESSERTS 215

Conclusion 222

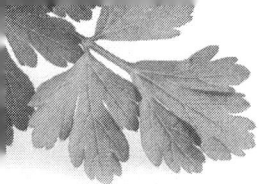

INTRODUCTION

Close your eyes for a moment and picture your skinny jeans. You know the pair we're talking about: those jeans you've had for longer than you'd care to admit (*cough cough* high school…) that you store deep in the corner of your closet as you longingly await for the day when you can once again slide into them without the use of Crisco or a decent car lubricant.

Well, if like us, your skinny jeans are collecting more dust than the old VHS player or Walkman you've hung on to for the last 15 years, you're not alone. No matter how hard we may try to lose weight and return to our thin figures of days long past, it never seems to be enough to bring those old and timeless jeans out retirement for an evening or two.

Ask anyone at your next New Year's Eve party what their #1 resolution is for the new year and you can count on hearing the same answer time and time again: to lose more weight. It's no surprise when you think about it really, especially when obesity is on a rise all around the world and fad diets seem to be more popular than ever before. Think about it: how many times have you clicked on the television late at night only to be bombarded with, "The latest! The greatest! The best darn diet you ever did see!" claiming to end your weight loss woes once and for all?

If only losing weight were that easy but, whether we'd like to admit it or not, there is no quick fix to weight loss. No amount of pills, waist trainers, or in-your-face 20 minute workouts will be enough to see real results so long as you're still snacking on a Big Mac or indulging in a bag of Oreos late at night.

Whether you are looking to lose weight for health reasons or just to look fabulous in your bikini on that upcoming beach vacation, you've come to the right place. Our recipes make it a breeze to incorporate the new Freestyle program into your busy lifestyle so you can see real (and lasting!) results for a happier, healthier you! Ready to get started? Let's jump right in!

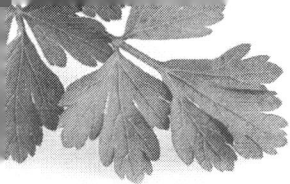

CHAPTER 1
A BRIEF HISTORY OF FREESTYLE

So, You Want to Lose a Little Weight, Huh?

The year is 1963. The setting? The loud-talkin', no-nonsense, bustling neighborhood of Queens, New York. The desires to lose weight? Pretty much the same as today, minus the convenience of counting calories with a clever app on your smart phone.

Desperate to the ease the complaints of women all around her crying for a better and safer way to lose weight, Jean Nidetch was determined to find a solution to this age-old problem. And find a solution she did.

When Jean Nidetch first set out to create Freestyle in the early 1960's, her goal was simple: to find an alternative to counting calories (if you think calorie counting is a headache now, imagine crunching the numbers in your head!). She also created a vibrant community where women could support each other in their weight loss journeys and, as the saying goes, the rest was history…

Old School Freestyle: An Overview

While the format of Freestyle has grown a bit over the years, the cornerstones remain the same. By combining a tried-and-true formula of points, meetings and exercise, Freestyle has been helping people all around the world get healthy and stay healthy for the better part of half a century!

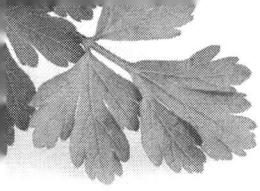

So, what exactly did old school Freestyle look like back in the day? We're glad you asked!

❖ **Point System**

Did you know that a single serving of salmon contains roughly 412 calories? How about the number of calories in a serving of cauliflower? Unless you're a certified nutritionist or a very skilled mathematician, it is nearly impossible to keep all of the calories in your favorite dishes straight! This is exactly why Freestyle created its popular point system. By assigning easy-to-remember points (think 5, 10, 15, 20, etc.) to the foods you eat, Freestyle makes it easy to keep track of your diet while subtly teaching you to eat better along the way (healthier foods are worth fewer points!).

❖ **In-Person Meetings**

For most of us, one of the biggest hurdles in weight loss is self-sabotage. Going it alone is a recipe for disaster, especially when those late night cravings kick in. That's why the folks at Freestyle came up with the in-person meetings that quickly made them a household name all around the world.

Back in the day, these meetings were pretty similar to the depictions you've seen on TV for the last decade or so (envision a crowded room lined with scales, cheerful employees, and no shortage of quirky name tags like "Baby Weight" and "Bikini Bod"). And, just like your favorite sitcom stars have done for decades, everyone would share their weight loss woes in a pseudo-Alcoholics Anonymous setting before carrying on with their day.

For a long time, these meetings served as one of the only ways to build a supportive, non-judgmental community in the weight loss industry. After all, this was an age long before social media or cell phones! Freestyle has adapted its meetings to meet the demands of the 21st century with its brand new Freestyle program, but more on that in a bit…

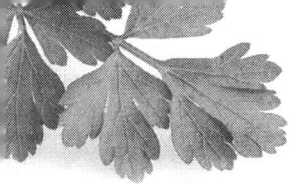

❖ Fitness and Exercise

The last (and one of the most important!) cornerstones of Freestyle is all about fitness, baby! Since its conception in the early 1960's, Freestyle has always advertised itself as more than a diet: it is a lifestyle. And like any healthy lifestyle, working out and exercising are a critical part of losing (and keeping off!) weight.

Unlike most diets that focus exclusively on the eating aspect of weight loss and nothing else, Freestyle has fitness points that are calculated into your daily point total. Not only does this take into account those hours spent sweating in the gym, it also helps you learn to enjoy exercising and, over time, live a healthier lifestyle!

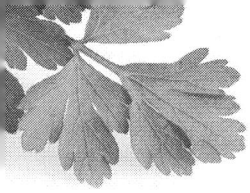

CHAPTER 2

A MODERN TWIST ON THE CLASSIC

What is the Freestyle Program?

Earning its claim to fame from none other than Oprah herself, the brand new Freestyle program is your first-class ticket to weight loss, 2018 style! Gone are the days of cumbersome points, awkward meetings, and embarrassing weigh-in's. With the new Freestyle program, you can enjoy all of the perks of the old school Freestyle program with these great new features:

- ➤ Zero Point Foods
- ➤ Virtual Health Coaching
- ➤ Online Resources
- ➤ Point Counting App
- ➤ In-Person or Virtual Meetings

What Sets the Freestyle Program Apart from Other Diets?

Unlike other diet programs available today, the Freestyle program was designed with the busy, modern dieter in mind! There is no need to clear out your freezer or schlep pounds of auto-delivery, pre-portioned meals into your kitchen each month since the Freestyle program allows you to cook with your own ingredients whenever you'd like. The best part? You will learn how

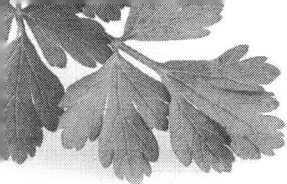

to prepare your own healthy meals (with no need to wean yourself off of those "fake" pre-portioned meals!).

Another great feature of the new Freestyle program is its dedication to building community to help you see real, lasting results. Whether you're interacting with your weight loss buddies online or chatting with your virtual coach, the Freestyle program makes it easy to find your pound-shedding tribe no matter where in the world your journey takes you!

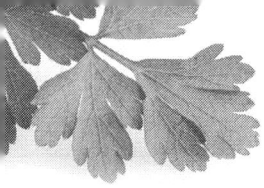

CHAPTER 3

ZERO POINT FOODS (NO, WE'RE NOT KIDDING!)

What are Zero Point Foods?

You read that right: the Freestyle program has a brand new list of zero point foods! Designed to help you explore (and grow to love!) healthier and heartier ingredients, these new zero points foods are a tasty way to give your body the nourishment it craves while still enjoying most of your favorite dishes!

Complete List of Zero Point Foods

Curious about what these zero point foods really look like on your plate? We've got you covered! Check out this complete list of ingredients, all of which are zero points in the new Freestyle program:

❖ Apples
❖ Applesauce
❖ Apricots
❖ Arrowroot
❖ Artichoke hearts
❖ Artichokes
❖ Arugula

❖ Asparagus
❖ Bamboo shoots
❖ Banana
❖ Beans
❖ Beets
❖ Berries
❖ Broccoli

❖ Broccoli rabe
❖ Broccoli slaw
❖ Broccolini
❖ Brussels sprouts
❖ Cabbage
❖ Calamari
❖ Cantaloupe

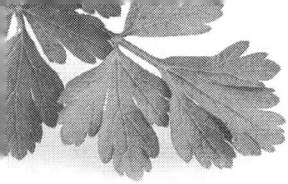

- ❖ Carrots
  - ❖ Cauliflower
  - ❖ Caviar (for those moments you're particularly fancy!)
  - ❖ Celery
  - ❖ Swiss chard
  - ❖ Cherries
  - ❖ Chicken breast (ground or tenderloin)
  - ❖ Clementine
  - ❖ Coleslaw
  - ❖ Collard greens
  - ❖ Corn
  - ❖ Cranberries
  - ❖ Cucumber
  - ❖ Daikon
  - ❖ Dates
  - ❖ Dragon fruit
  - ❖ Edamame
  - ❖ Egg substitutes
  - ❖ Egg whites
  - ❖ Eggs (whole)
  - ❖ Endive
  - ❖ Fennel
  - ❖ Figs
  - ❖ Fish
  - ❖ Fish fillet
  - ❖ Fruit cocktail

- ❖ Fruit cup
  - ❖ Fruit salad
  - ❖ Fruit (unsweetened)
  - ❖ Garlic
  - ❖ Ginger root
  - ❖ Grapefruit
  - ❖ Grapes
  - ❖ Greens
  - ❖ Guavas
  - ❖ Hearts of Palm
  - ❖ Hominy
  - ❖ Honeydew melon
  - ❖ Jackfruit
  - ❖ Jerk chicken breast
  - ❖ Jerusalem artichokes
  - ❖ Jicama (yam bean)
  - ❖ Kiwi
  - ❖ Kohlrabi
  - ❖ Kumquats
  - ❖ Leeks
  - ❖ Lemon
  - ❖ Lemon zest
  - ❖ Lentils
  - ❖ Lettuce
  - ❖ Lime
  - ❖ Lime zest
  - ❖ Litchis
  - ❖ Mangoes
  - ❖ Melon
  - ❖ Meng bean sprouts

- ❖ Mung dal
  - ❖ Mushrooms
  - ❖ Nectarine
  - ❖ Nori seaweed
  - ❖ Okra
  - ❖ Onions
  - ❖ Oranges
  - ❖ Papaya
  - ❖ Parsley
  - ❖ Passion fruit
  - ❖ Pea shoots
  - ❖ Peaches
  - ❖ Pea pods (black eye)
  - ❖ Pears
  - ❖ Peas and carrots
  - ❖ Misc. peas
  - ❖ Peppers
  - ❖ Pepperoncini
  - ❖ Persimmons
  - ❖ Pickles
  - ❖ Pico de gallo
  - ❖ Pimientos (canned)
  - ❖ Pineapple
  - ❖ Plumcots
  - ❖ Plums
  - ❖ Pomegranate seeds
  - ❖ Pomegranates
  - ❖ Pomelo (pummelo)
  - ❖ Pumpkin
  - ❖ Pumpkin puree

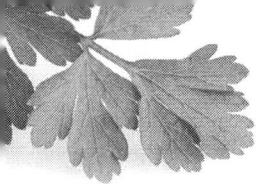

- ❖ Radicchio
- ❖ Radishes
- ❖ Raspberries
- ❖ Rutabagas
- ❖ Salad
- ❖ Salsa verde
- ❖ Salsa (fat-free)
- ❖ Sashimi
- ❖ Satay (chicken, without peanut sauce)
- ❖ Satsuma (mandarin)
- ❖ Sauerkraut
- ❖ Scallions
- ❖ Seaweed
- ❖ Shallots
- ❖ Shellfish
- ❖ Spinach
- ❖ Sprouts (including alfalfa beans and lentils)
- ❖ Summer squash (including zucchini)
- ❖ Winter squash (including spaghetti squash)
- ❖ Starfruit
- ❖ Strawberries
- ❖ Succotash
- ❖ Tangelo
- ❖ Tangerines
- ❖ Taro
- ❖ Tofu
- ❖ Tomatillos
- ❖ Tomatoes
- ❖ Turkey breast (ground or sirloin)
- ❖ Turnips
- ❖ Vegetable stick
- ❖ Mixed vegetables
- ❖ Stir fry vegetables
- ❖ Water chestnuts
- ❖ Water crests
- ❖ Watermelon
- ❖ Yogurt (Greek, plain, or soy)

CHAPTER 4

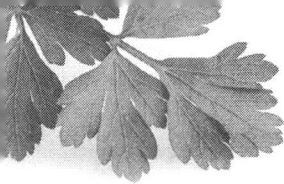

WORKING OUT ON
THE FREESTYLE DIET

Fitness Points

Just like the original Freestyle program, Freestyle incorporates exercise and fitness into your weight loss journey! By keeping track of your food points and fitness points in one, easy-to-use app, the new Freestyle program makes it easy to track everything from steps to cardio workouts, and everything in between!

The best part? If you have an iPhone or smart watch, the Freestyle app will sync right with your other tracking software so everything stays organized and in one accessible place!

It's All About Variety!

Ever heard the saying, "variety is the spice of life?" Well, when it comes to workout routines, variety is the key to your success! Ask any gym guru about their secret to gaining muscle and losing fat, and they will tell you that mixing up workouts and trying new activities keeps things fun and exciting (not to mention can curtail those, "But I really don't want to go to the gym today!" feelings we all have every now and then).

Need a little inspiration? Check out this sample beginner weekly routine that incorporates a bit of everything for a well-rounded and engaging workout:

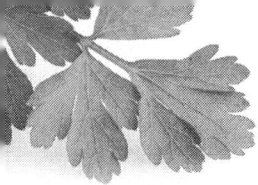

- ➢ **Monday:** Cardio! Start your week with a fresh burst of energy by going for a run (or walk) around the neighborhood.

- ➢ **Tuesday:** Weight training! Hit the gym for some bicep curls and leg presses or, if you have the equipment at home, fit in a few sets during a commercial break or two while you catch up with your DVR recordings.

- ➢ **Wednesday:** Yoga or Pilates! Whether you're looking to slow down a bit with some restorative yoga or fire up your core with a set of Pilates 100's, this day is all about building muscle in a fun, alternative way.

- ➢ **Thursday:** Zumba or Dancing (otherwise known as "super fun cardio")! Try out a Zumba class or DVD at home, or just crank up the tunes and enjoy a 20-minute dance party in your living room. You'll be shocked how much fat you can burn when you're busy dancing the blues away!

- ➢ **Friday:** Rest (you've earned it!).

- ➢ **Saturday:** Jogging or Walking! Nothing starts the weekend off right quite like a relaxing jog or stroll around the block on a Saturday morning. Treat your heart to a relaxing yet energetic workout as you ease into the weekend state of mind.

- ➢ **Sunday:** Slow things down with some targeted resistance training! Try a few sets of push-ups or sit-ups, squats, or even work with resistance bands.

No matter which workout you choose to incorporate into your lifestyle with the new Freestyle diet, you'll find that this healthy, new you is here to stay. The best part? The longer you work out and meet your daily fitness point goals, the easier it will be to make your way to the gym every day and, dare we say, maybe start enjoying a good workout along the way?!

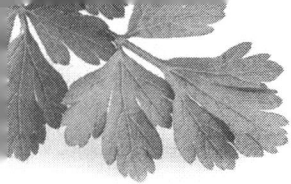

CHAPTER 5

EAT WHAT YOU WANT, WHERE YOU WANT!

Freestyle On the Go

One of the best perks of working with our recipes and the Freestyle diet is the ease by which you can take any of these dishes with you on the go! Whether you're bouncing back and forth between soccer practice and theater try-outs, trying to fit a healthy lunch break in between meetings, or whipping up something quick after a long day at the office, our innovative recipes use Freestyle-friendly foods to turn your favorite meals into hearty dishes your whole family will love.

Food Prepping: A Beginner's Guide

New to meal prepping? We recommend setting aside one day per week to prepare a recipe or two (or three!) and portioning everything out into grab n' go containers for the week ahead! Not only will you be able to enjoy a healthy meal in a pinch, you'll also learn to carve out some time to make your weight loss journey a priority for years to come! If you're unsure where exactly to start, check out our no-nonsense reference guide to Meal Prepping 101 below:

> ➤ **Containers:** Start by selecting a week's worth of sturdy, reliable food storage containers (preferably leak-proof and dishwasher-safe for easy cleaning).

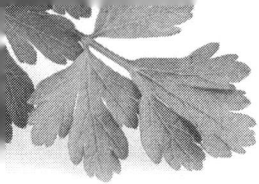

➢ **Prep like a conveyor belt:** Lay out all of your empty containers in a neat row or two and add finished dishes in as you go. All set with the chicken breasts? Toss one in a container. Are the steamed veggies ready to go? Divvy them up into each container. Continue like this until your completed meal has been replicated for the entire week!

➢ **Clear out a shelf:** Unless you're absolutely positive that you will eat your meals on each day of the coming week, we recommend clearing off a shelf in your freezer so your fresh cooked masterpieces last as long as you need! Hint: wrap your food containers in plastic wrap or pop them in a freezer-safe re-sealable bag to avoid freezer burn.

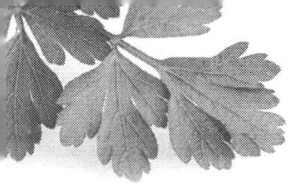

CHAPTER 6

LIVING THE FREESTYLE LIFESTYLE

Living a Healthy Life vs. a "Skinny" Life

If you've ever flipped through one of the tabloids at the checkout counter or browsed celebrity gossip sites online, you know that there seems to be a bit of confusion between the concepts of *healthy* and *skinny*. All too often, we mistake skinniness for overall health or a smaller dress size for wellbeing. This mindset is exactly why fad diets became an overnight international craze (and, undoubtedly, why quick fix procedures seem to be more popular than living a healthy lifestyle).

The new Freestyle program is challenging this thought pattern though, and instead challenges you to live an overall healthier lifestyle. By encouraging you to try out hearty ingredients like those found in the zero points list or rewarding you for earning fitness points, the Freestyle program was designed to teach you healthier habits so, in turn, you can see the results you've always craved when looking in the mirror.

Sharing the Freestyle Program with Your Loved Ones

By emphasizing the importance of community in weight loss, the Freestyle diet encourages you to share your new-found love of healthy eating with those around you. In the same light, our recipes have been designed to share so your entire family can get in on the fun and start living a healthier, happier lifestyle together!

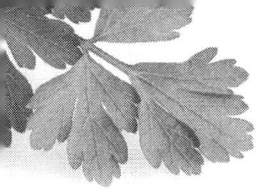

Still hesitant about signing up for the new Freestyle program by yourself? Try it with a friend! Whether you're simply testing out a new recipe for girl's night or taking the plunge of signing up for the program with your spouse, losing weight can actually be fun when you partner up with a loved one!

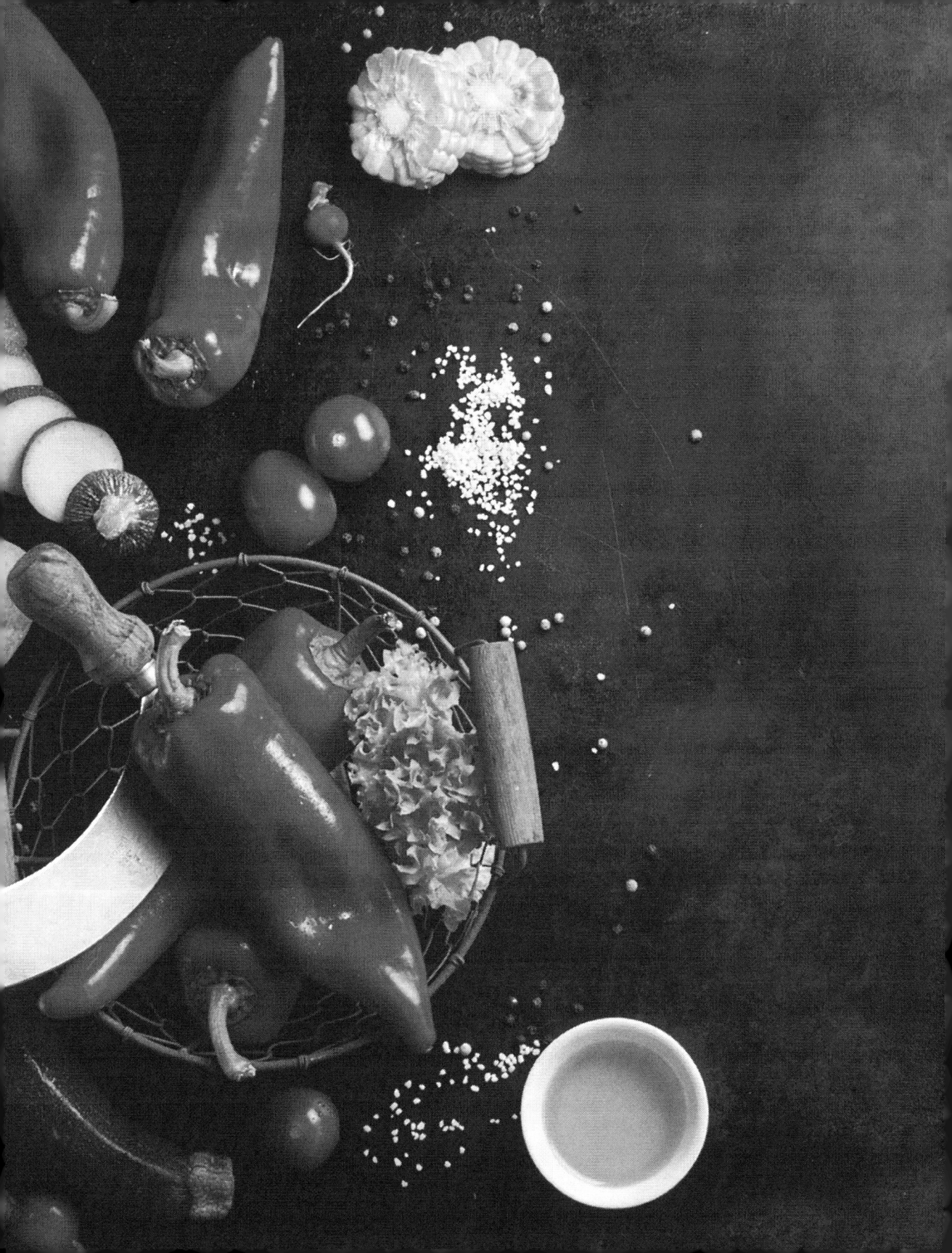

BREAKFASTS

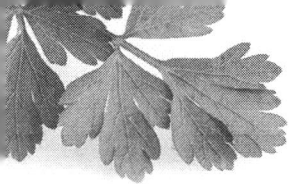

Brownie Batter Oats

(Prep Time: 8 HOUR 5 MIN | Cook Time: N/A | Serves: 1)

Ingredients:

For oats:

½ cup fat-free plain Greek
yogurt

½ cup almond milk
(unsweetened)

2 tbsp Dutch-process cocoa
powder

1 ripe banana (peeled, mashed)

½ cup oats

Pinch kosher salt

Directions:

1. Add all ingredients to a resealable jar/container and stir to combine. Seal and chill overnight.
2. When ready to serve, stir once or twice to recombine and enjoy.

Freestyle SmartPoints Per Serving: 4

(Calories 365 | Total Fats 5g | Net Carbs: 54g | Protein 20g | Fiber: 11g)

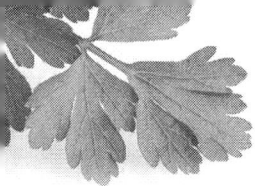

Café Mocha Breakfast Smoothie

(Prep Time: 5 MIN | Cook Time: N/A | Serves: 2)

Ingredients:

For smoothie:

½ frozen banana

2 Medjool dates (pitted)

1 ½ tbsp cacao powder

½ cup spinach

1 tbsp chia seeds

3 ice cubes

¼ avocado (peeled, pitted)

½ cup strongly brewed coffee (coffee)

⅓ cup almond milk

Directions:

1. Add all ingredients to a blender and blitz until smooth and lump-free.
2. Pour into two glasses and enjoy immediately*.

*To feel fuller longer, enjoy at room temperature.

Freestyle SmartPoints Per Serving: 9

(Calories 202 | Total Fats 6g | Net Carbs: 27g | Protein 6g | Fiber: 9g)

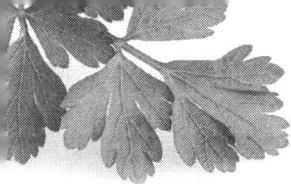

Chia Seed and Mango Breakfast Pudding

(Prep Time: 5 HOUR 10 MIN | Cook Time: N/A | Serves: 1)

Ingredients:

For pudding:

¼ cup chia seeds

1 cup almond milk

¼ tsp cinnamon

½ tsp vanilla essence

½ tsp frozen mango

1 tbsp coconut milk

1 tsp goji berries (to garnish)

1 tsp coconut flakes (to garnish)

Directions:

1. Combine the chia seeds with the almond milk, cinnamon, and vanilla essence in a large jug and allow to rest for 4-5 hours, until the mixture becomes a gel-like consistency.

2. In a food blender, process the mango and coconut milk to a smooth puree.

3. Pour the mango-coconut mixture into the bottom of a tall serving glass, and using a small spoon lay the chia pudding carefully on top.

4. Garnish with goji berries and coconut flakes.

Freestyle SmartPoints Per Serving: 10

(Calories 401 | Total Fats 21g | Net Carbs: 15g | Protein 15g | Fiber: 22g)

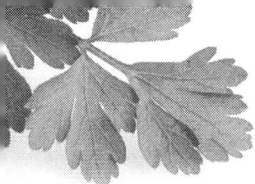

Fruit and Honey Breakfast Quinoa

(Prep Time: 5 MIN | Cook Time: 15 MIN | Serves: 1)

Ingredients:

For quinoa:
½ cup almond milk

¼ cup quinoa

1 tbsp organic honey

For topping:
1 cup fresh mixed fruit
(chopped)

Directions:

1. Add the milk to a small saucepan and bring to a boil, add the quinoa and stir. Cover the pan with a lid and turn the heat down to moderately low. Cook for approximately 15 minutes until the milk is completely absorbed.
2. Take off the heat and stir in the organic honey until incorporated.
3. Transfer to a serving bowl and top with fresh fruit.

Freestyle SmartPoints Per Serving: 7

(Calories 350 | Total Fats 3g | Net Carbs: 60g | Protein 11g | Fiber: 7g)

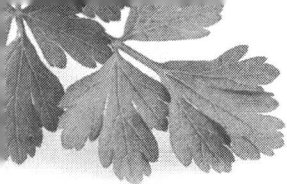

Butternut Squash and Sausage Breakfast Bake

(Prep Time: 10 MIN | Cook Time: 30 MIN | Serves: 4)

Ingredients:

For cooking:
Nonstick spray

For bake:
1 pound lean breakfast turkey
sausage (ground)
2 tsp olive oil
½ medium red onion (peeled,
finely chopped)
2 cups butternut squash
(peeled, seeded, finely
chopped)
4 cups fresh spinach (roughly
chopped)
4 medium eggs
Whites of 4 medium eggs

Seasoning:
½ tsp kosher salt
½ tsp powdered garlic
½ tsp dried oregano
½ tsp black pepper

Directions:

1. Preheat the main oven to 400 degrees F. Spritz a small casserole dish with nonstick spray and set to one side.
2. Sauté the ground sausage in a large skillet over moderately high heat. Break up the meat using a wooden spoon as it cooks, until browned. Set the cooked sausage to one side.
3. To the same hot skillet, add the oil. Add the red onion and butternut squash, sauté for several minutes until softened and tender. If the mixture catches, add a drop of water.
4. Sprinkle with the seasoning and stir well.
5. Add the chopped spinach, cook for a couple of minutes until wilted.
6. In a small bowl, whisk together the whole eggs and egg whites.
7. Transfer the butternut squash mixture to the casserole dish, scatter with the cooked sausage. Slowly and evenly, pour the eggs over the mixture.
8. Place in the oven and bake for just over 25 minutes, until the egg has set completely.
9. Slice into squares and serve hot/warm.

Freestyle Smart Points Per Serving: 6

(Calories 331 | Total Fats 16g | Net Carbs: 9g | Protein 33g | Fiber: 3g)

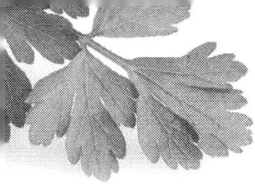

Cheesy Egg and Bacon Breakfast Muffins

(Prep Time: 15 MIN | Cook Time: 20 MIN | Serves: 6)

Ingredients:

For cooking:
Nonstick spray

For muffins:
6 rashers turkey bacon
(chopped)
1 medium zucchini (finely
chopped)
¼ cup skim milk
6 medium eggs
Whites of 6 medium eggs
½ cup semi-skim mozzarella
cheese (shredded)

Seasoning:
Sea salt and black pepper

Directions:

1. Preheat the main oven to 375 degrees F. Spritz a 6-hole muffin tin with nonstick spray and set to one side.
2. Spritz a skillet with nonstick spray. Add the turkey bacon and sauté over moderate heat until crispy. Remove from the skillet and set to one side. Drain away any bacon fat.
3. To the same hot skillet add the chopped zucchini. Sauté for 3-4 minutes, until softened. Take off the heat and set to one side.
4. Whisk together the milk, whole eggs, egg whites, and seasoning in a mixing bowl, until the eggs froth. Add the cooked bacon, zucchini, and mozzarella to the egg mixture. Stir to combine.
5. Pour the mixture equally into the prepared muffin tin.
6. Place in the oven and cook for 20 minutes, until completely set.
7. Enjoy warm.

Freestyle Smart Points Per Serving: 2

(Calories 145 | Total Fats 8g | Net Carbs: 2g | Protein 14g | Fiber: 1g

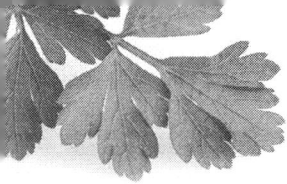

Choc Chip Banana Breakfast Bars

(Prep Time: 15 MIN | Cook Time: N/A | Serves: 9)

Ingredients:

For bars:

⅓ cup organic crunchy peanut butter

2 medium, ripe bananas (peeled, mashed)

1 tsp ground cinnamon

2 tbsp maple syrup

½ cup flaxseed meal

2 cups rolled oats

2 tbsp chia seeds

¼ cup shredded coconut (unsweetened)

⅓ cup semisweet choc chips

Directions:

1. Line an 8" square baking dish with parchment paper, set to one side.
2. In a mixing bowl, combine the peanut butter, mashed banana, cinnamon, and maple syrup.
3. Add the flaxseed meal, rolled oats, chia seeds, and coconut. Mix until well combined.
4. Fold in the choc chips until evenly distributed.
5. Press the mixture into the baking dish, ensuring it reaches into all of the corners.
6. Chill for 3 hours. Slice into 9 equal squares and enjoy.
7. Keep chilled.

Freestyle Smart Points Per Serving: 8

(Calories 249 | Total Fats 13g | Net Carbs: 22g | Protein 7g | Fiber: 7g)

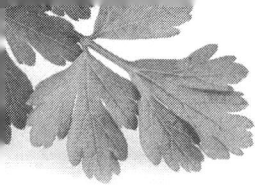

Ham and Apple Swiss Cheese Melts

(Prep Time: 10 MIN | Cook Time: 10 MIN | Serves: 6)

Ingredients:

For mustard sauce:

1½ tsp Worcestershire sauce

1½ tbsp Dijon mustard

½ tsp brown sugar

For melts:

3 reduced-fat multigrain
English muffins (halved)

2 apples (cored, thinly sliced)

12 ounces deli ham (sliced)

6 slices low-fat Swiss cheese

Directions:

1. Preheat the main oven to 350 degrees F.
2. In a small bowl, combine the Worcestershire sauce, Dijon mustard, and brown sugar. Spread the mixture evenly onto each muffin half.
3. Arrange the muffin halves on a baking sheet (cut-side up).
4. Top each muffin with an equal amount of sliced apple, followed by 2 ounces of sliced deli ham, and finally a slice of cheese.
5. Place in the oven and cook for several minutes until the cheese melts.
6. Enjoy hot.

Freestyle Smart Points Per Serving: 5

(Calories 270 | Total Fats 12.5g | Net Carbs: 13.5g | Protein 22g | Fiber: 6g)

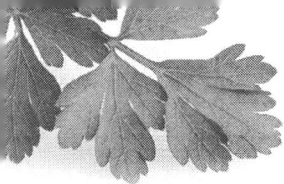

Lemon and Blueberry Waffles

(Prep Time: 10 MIN | Cook Time: 10 MIN | Serves: 3)

Ingredients:

For cooking:

Nonstick spray

For waffles:

1 medium egg

¾ cup skim milk

¼ cup applesauce (unsweetened)

2 tbsp lemon juice

1 tsp vanilla essence

1 tsp lemon zest (grated)

1 tbsp granulated sugar

2 tsp baking powder

1 cup flour

¾ cup frozen/fresh blueberries

Directions:

1. Preheat your waffle iron.
2. In a large jug, whisk up the egg until it froths.
3. Beat in the milk, applesauce, lemon juice, and vanilla essence.
4. Stir in the lemon zest, sugar, baking powder, and flour until the mixture is relatively lump-free.
5. Finally, fold in the blueberries.
6. Spritz the waffle iron with nonstick spray.
7. Cook a ⅓ of a cup of batter in the waffle iron at a time (for approximately 7-8 minutes).
8. Enjoy warm.

Freestyle Smart Points Per Serving: 7

(Calories 224 | Total Fats 2.8g | Net Carbs: 38g | Protein 7g | Fiber: 6g)

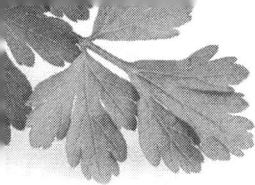

Country Cottage Pancakes

(Prep Time: 10 MIN | Cook Time: 15 MIN | Serves: 4)

Ingredients:

For cooking:

Nonstick spray

For pancakes:

1 cup low-fat cottage cheese

8 medium eggs

4 tbsp almond flour

4 tbsp coconut flour

½ tsp bicarb of soda

1 tsp lemon zest (grated)

Pinch kosher salt

½ tsp vanilla essence

4 tbsp sweetened almond milk

Directions:

1. Add all ingredients (excluding the almond milk) to a blender and blitz until smooth.

2. Spritz a skillet with nonstick spray and place over moderately high heat.

3. Ladle a ¼ cup of batter at a time into the skillet. When the mixture begins to bubble, flip and cook until the bubbles start to pop and the edges are firm and cooked.

4. Repeat with the remaining batter and serve straight away.

Freestyle Smart Points Per Serving: 3

(Calories 265 | Total Fats 15g | Net Carbs: 5g | Protein 23g | Fiber: 3g)

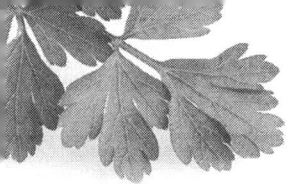

Make-Ahead Breakfast Muffin Sandwiches

(Prep Time: 10 MIN | Cook Time: 15 MIN | Serves: 12)

Ingredients:

For cooking:
Nonstick spray

For sandwiches:
3 cups liquid egg substitute
Kosher salt and black pepper
12 rashers centre-cut bacon
12 lower-calorie English breakfast muffins (halved)
12 low-fat American cheese slices

Directions:

1. Preheat the main oven to 350 degrees F. Spritz a 13x9" baking tray generously with nonstick spray.
2. Pour the egg substitute into the tray and season with kosher salt and black pepper, stir well and place in the oven for 15 minutes until cooked and set.
3. While the eggs cook, fry the rashers of bacon.
4. When the eggs are finished cooking, slice them into 12 equal squares. Set the bacon and eggs aside to cool completely.
5. Fill each muffin with one square of egg, one rasher of bacon, and one slice of cheese.
6. Wrap each muffin tightly in foil and place in a large Ziploc bag. Seal the bag and pop in the freezer for up to 90 days.
7. When ready to serve; allow to thaw at room temperature overnight. The following morning, warm in the microwave for 60-70 seconds and enjoy.

Freestyle Smart Points Per Serving: 4

(Calories 160 | Total Fats 1.5g | Net Carbs: 18g | Protein 16g | Fiber: 6g)

INSTANT POT BREAKFASTS

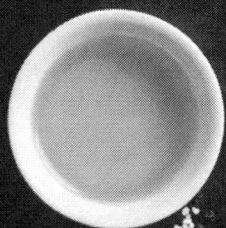

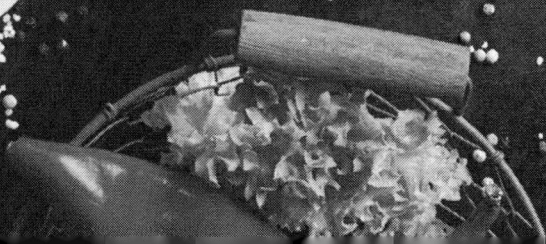

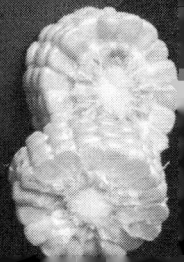

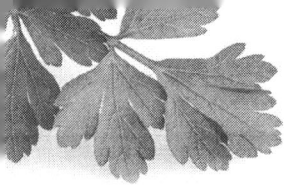

Scrambled Eggs with Salmon

(Prep Time: 15 MIN | Cook Time: 10 MIN | Serves: 4)

Ingredients:

For cooking:

1 tbsp olive oil

1 cup fish stock

For scrambled eggs:

7oz salmon fillet

4 eggs

2 spring onions, finely chopped

1 leek, chopped

2 garlic cloves, crushed

Seasoning:

1 tsp salt

1 tbsp fresh dill

½ tsp red pepper flakes

Directions:

1. Plug in the Instant Pot and pour in the fish stock in the inner pot. Add salmon and sprinkle with some salt.

2. Seal the lid and set the steam release handle to the Sealing position. Press the Manual button and set the timer for 5 minutes on High pressure.

3. When done, perform a quick pressure release and open the lid. Remove the salmon and transfer to a cutting board. Using a sharp knife, chop the fillet into bite-sized pieces and set aside.

4. Now, press the Sauté button. Heat up the oil and add leeks and garlic. Cook for 4-5 minutes, stirring constantly.

5. Add spring onions and chopped salmon. Season with more salt and pepper. Give it a good stir and continue to cook for another 5 minutes.

6. Finally, add eggs and stir all well. Cook for 1-2 minutes.

7. Remove from the pot and sprinkle with fresh dill. Serve immediately.

Freestyle SmartPoints Per Serving: 5

(Calories 187 | Total Fats 11.5g | Net Carbs: 3.9g | Protein 17.1g | Fiber: 0.6g)

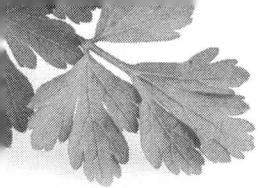

Trout Brussels Sprout Hash

(Prep Time: 15 MIN | Cook Time: 15 MIN | Serves: 6)

Ingredients:

For cooking:
2 tsp butter

For hash:
1 lb trout fillets, cut into bite-sized pieces

1 lb Brussels sprouts, chopped

2 medium-sized carrots, chopped

1 large turnip, chopped

3 large eggs

Seasoning:
1 tsp sea salt

1 tsp dried parsley, ground

¼ tsp dried dill, ground

½ tsp Italian seasoning

Directions:

1. Plug in the Instant Pot and place butter in the stainless steel insert. Press the Saute button and gently stir, until butter melts.
2. Add chopped trout and sprinkle with some salt. Cook for 3-4 minutes, stirring occasionally.
3. Now, add Brussels sprouts, carrots, and turnips. Add water enough to cover and sprinkle with dried parsley, dill, and Italian seasoning. Stir well and close the lid. Set the steam release handle and press the Manual button. Set the timer for 7 minutes and cook on High pressure.
4. When you hear the cookers end signal, perform a quick pressure release and open the pot. Drain the ingredients and return to the pot.
5. Press the Sauté button and poach the eggs on top. Cook for 2 more minutes, or until the eggs are set.
6. Transfer all to a serving plate and enjoy!

Freestyle SmartPoints Per Serving: 6

(Calories 240 | Total Fats 10.5g | Net Carbs: 8.9g | Protein 26.3g | Fiber: 3.9g)

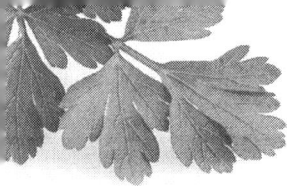

Mushroom Pepper Quiche

(Prep Time: 15 MIN | Cook Time: 17 MIN | Serves: 6)

Ingredients:

For cooking:
2 tsp olive oil

For quiche:
2 cups button mushrooms, sliced

1 large red bell pepper, chopped

1 large green bell pepper, diced

2 cups fresh spinach, chopped

6 eggs, beaten

¼ cup milk, fat-free

Seasoning:
1 tsp sea salt

½ tsp black pepper, ground

1 tsp dried thyme, ground

Directions:

1. Line a fitting spring-form pan with some parchment paper and grease the walls with some cooking spray. Set aside.
2. Plug in the Instant Pot and grease the stainless steel insert with olive oil. Add mushrooms and bell peppers. Cook for 3-4 minutes, stirring occasionally.
3. Add spinach and continue to cook for 3 more minutes or until spinach is wilted. Transfer all to a prepared spring-form pan.
4. In a large mixing bowl, combine eggs, and remaining spices. Lightly whisk and pour over the vegetables.
5. Add 1 cup of water to the pot and set the trivet on the bottom. Place the pan on top and securely lock the lid.
6. Set the steam release handle by moving the valve to the Sealing position. Press the Manual button and cook for 10 minutes on High pressure.
7. When done, perform a quick pressure release and open the pot. Carefully transfer the pan to a wire rack and let it chill for a while.
8. Optionally, sprinkle with some chives before serving. Enjoy!

Freestyle SmartPoints Per Serving: 3

(Calories 101 | Total Fats 6.4g | Net Carbs: 4g | Protein 7.3g | Fiber: 1g)

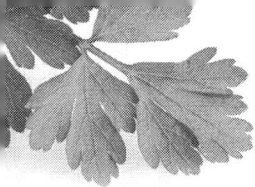

Pumpkin Breakfast Bowl

(Prep Time: 15 MIN | Cook Time: 20 MIN | Serves: 2)

Ingredients:

For cooking:
Coconut oil cooking spray

For pumpkin bowl:
1 lb sweet pumpkin, cut into small cubes

1 large red bell pepper, cut into bite-sized pieces

1 tsp cayenne pepper, ground

¼ tsp red chili pepper flakes

1 tsp salt

½ tsp garlic powder

For sauce:
1 cup cherry tomatoes, diced

1 tbsp tomato paste

1 tsp dried oregano, ground

½ tsp onion powder

1 tsp fresh parsley, finely chopped

1 tsp salt

¼ tsp black pepper, ground

Directions:

1. Combine all sauce ingredients in a food processor or a blender. Pulse until smooth and creamy. Set aside.
2. Plug in the Instant Pot and place pumpkin and bell peppers in the stainless steel insert. Sprinkle with cayenne pepper, chili, salt, and garlic powder. Stir well and add water enough to cover all ingredients. Securely lock the lid and set the steam release handle. Press the Manual button and set the timer for 4 minutes. Cook on High pressure.
3. When you hear the cookers end signal, perform a quick pressure release and open the pot. Let it chill for a while.
4. Meanwhile, preheat the oven to 375 degrees. Line some parchment paper over a small baking sheet. Transfer the vegetable mixture and spread evenly over the baking sheet. Drizzle all with sauce and bake for 8-10 minutes.
5. Transfer into serving bowls, and optionally, top with fat-free Greek yogurt and sliced avocado.

Freestyle SmartPoints Per Serving: 3

(Calories 74 | Total Fats 0.6g | Net Carbs: 15g | Protein 3g | Fiber: 2.7g)

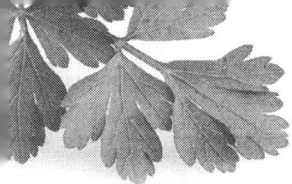

Green Pea Tomato Omelette

(Prep Time: 5 MIN | Cook Time: 10 MIN | Serves: 2)

Ingredients:

For cooking:
2 tsp butter

For omelette:
6 large eggs

½ cup green peas

1 large Roma tomato, finely chopped

1 tbsp fresh parsley, finely chopped

Seasoning:
1 tsp fresh dill, finely chopped

½ tsp fresh thyme, finely chopped

¼ tsp dried oregano, ground

1 tsp salt

Directions:

1. In a large mixing bowl, whisk the eggs along with fresh dill, thyme, and oregano. Set aside.
2. Plug in the Instant Pot and place the beans and tomato in the stainless steel insert. Sprinkle with parsley and some salt to taste. Stir well and pour in ½ cup of water. Securely lock the lid. Set the steam release handle and press the Manual button. Set the timer for 7 minutes and cook on High pressure.
3. When done, perform a quick release of the pressure and open the pot. Remove contents and set aside.
4. Now, melt the butter in the stainless steel insert using Sauté heat. Pour in the egg mixture and cook for 2-3 minutes, or until set.
5. Turn off the pot and transfer the omelet to a serving plate. Spoon the vegetable mixture on one half. Fold the other half and serve immediately.

Freestyle SmartPoints Per Serving: 5

(Calories 149 | Total Fats 9.6g | Net Carbs: 4g | Protein 11g | Fiber: 1.5g)

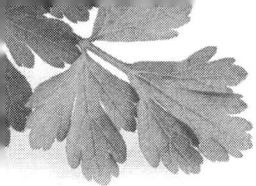

Salmon Spinach Muffins

(Prep Time: 15 MIN | Cook Time: 20 MIN | Serves: 6)

Ingredients:

For cooking:
Cooking spray

For muffins:
1 lb fresh spinach, chopped

6 oz salmon fillets, cut into bite-sized pieces

6 large eggs

1 cup celery leaves, finely chopped

2 tbsp all-purpose flour

1 tsp baking powder

Seasoning:
1 tsp Italian seasoning

½ tsp sea salt

½ tsp black pepper, ground

¼ tsp dried rosemary, ground

Directions:

1. In a large mixing bowl, combine all ingredients along with seasoning. Mix until well incorporated.
2. Spoon the mixture into silicone muffin molds greased with cooking spray.
3. Plug in the Instant Pot and pour 1 cup of water into the stainless steel insert. Position a trivet in the pot and set the molds on top.
4. Securely lock the lid and adjust the steam release handle by moving the valve to the Sealing position.
5. Press the Manual button and set the timer for 20 minutes. Cook on High pressure.
6. When you hear the cookers end signal, perform a quick pressure release by moving the valve to the Venting position.
7. Open the pot and carefully transfer the muffins to a wire rack using oven mitts.
8. Let cool for a while before serving.

Freestyle SmartPoints Per Serving: 4

(Calories 248 | Total Fats 7.1g | Net Carbs: 6g | Protein 14.3g | Fiber: 2g)

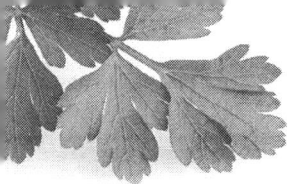

Breakfast Mushroom Tortillas

(Prep Time: 10 MIN | Cook Time: 12 MIN | Serves: 5)

Ingredients:

For cooking:
Nonstick cooking spray
1 cup chicken broth

For mushrooms:
1 cup button mushrooms, sliced
4 large eggs
1 tbsp skim milk
1 tbsp Parmesan cheese, grated
1 tbsp fresh parsley, finely chopped
5 wholewheat tortillas

Seasoning:
½ tsp fresh mint, finely chopped
¼ tsp garlic powder
¼ tsp red chili flakes
¼ tsp salt

Directions:

1. In a large mixing bowl, combine eggs, milk, cheese, and parsley. Whisk until well combined and set aside.
2. Plug in the Instant Pot pour the chicken broth in the stainless steel insert. Sprinkle with some garlic powder, salt, and red chili flakes. Securely lock the lid and adjust the steam release handle.
3. Press the Manual button and set the timer for 8 minutes. Cook on High pressure.
4. When you hear the cookers ending signal, perform a quick pressure release and open the pot. Drain the mushrooms and remove the liquid.
5. Pour in the egg mixture and add drained mushrooms. Stir well and press the Sauté button. Cook for 3-4 minutes, or until the eggs are set.
6. Divide the mixture between 5 tortillas and wrap. Secure with a toothpick and serve immediately. Enjoy!

Freestyle SmartPoints Per Serving: 5

(Calories 188 | Total Fats 5.9g | Net Carbs: 20.1g | Protein 11.5g | Fiber: 3.2g)

POULTRY

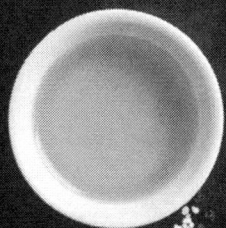
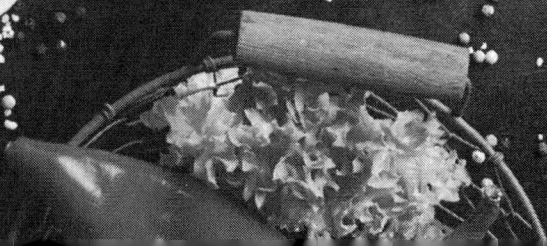
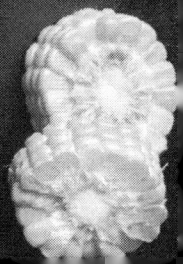

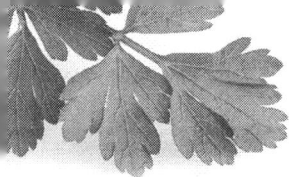

Asian Style Chicken & Cashews

(Prep Time: 5 MIN | Cook Time: 20 MIN | Serves: 4)

Ingredients:

For cooking:
Nonstick spray

For chicken:
1⅓ pounds skinless, boneless chicken breast (chopped)

Olive oil (to toss)

½ tsp black pepper

16 ounces Chinese vegetable mix

¼ cup cashews

For sauce:
⅓ cup low-salt soy sauce

⅓ cup water

2 tbsp hoisin sauce

2 tbsp runny honey

1 tbsp Chinese garlic chili paste

2 garlic cloves (peeled, minced)

1 tbsp cornstarch

Directions:

1. Preheat the main oven to 400 degrees F. Line a baking sheet with aluminum foil and spritz with nonstick spray.
2. Spritz the chicken breast with cooking spray and gently toss with olive oil. Season with pepper.
3. Arrange the chicken in a single layer on the prepared baking sheet. Cook in the preheated oven for 10 minutes.
4. In the meantime, combine all of the sauce ingredients in a pan. Bring to boil, before reducing the heat to a simmer. Cook for between 4-6 minutes, until the mixture can easily coat the back of a spoon. Do not allow the sauce to burn.
5. Remove the chicken from the oven.
6. Add the mixed vegetables and cashews.
7. Drizzle with the sauce and toss well to coat evenly.
8. Return the pan to the oven and cook until the veggies are tender but crisp; 8-10 minutes. Serve.

Freestyle SmartPoints Per Serving: 5

(Calories 326 | Total Fats 6g | Net Carbs: 23g | Protein 37g | Fiber: 4g)

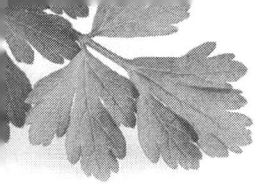

Asian Turkey Burgers with Spicy Slaw

(Prep Time: 15 MIN | Cook Time: 10 MIN | Serves: 4)

Ingredients:

For cooking:

Nonstick spray

For slaw:

2 cups mixed shredded cabbage

3 tsp Asian hot sauce

½ cup fat-free mayo

1 tbsp rice vinegar

2 tsp fresh cilantro (minced)

2 tsp fresh chives (minced)

½ tsp salt

½ tsp brown sugar

For burgers:

1 pound ground turkey

1 tbsp soy sauce

2 tsp grated fresh ginger

2 tsp minced garlic

4 whole grain burger buns (toasted)

Directions:

1. Add all of the slaw ingredients to a bowl and mix until combined. Set aside while you prepare the burgers.
2. Add all of the burger ingredients (excluding the burger buns) to a second bowl and mix, using clean hands, until combined.
3. Divide and shape the mixture into 4 equal patties.
4. Grill the patties for approximately 4 minutes on each side, until thoroughly cooked through.
5. Arrange the cooked burgers in the buns and top each with the prepared slaw.

Freestyle SmartPoints Per Serving: 9

(Calories 320 | Total Fats 10.5g | Net Carbs: 23.5g | Protein 27g | Fiber: 5g)

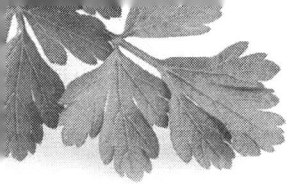

Baked Apricot and Olive Chicken in Wine

(Prep Time: 8 HOUR 10 MIN | Cook Time: 55 MIN | Serves: 6)

Ingredients:

For chicken:

¾ cup green olives

2 pounds boneless, skinless chicken thighs

⅓ cup dried apricots (roughly chopped)

5 cloves garlic (peeled, minced)

For marinade:

⅓ cup sherry vinegar

2 tbsp olive oil

1½ tbsp oregano

For wine:

2 tbsp brown sugar

½ cup dry white wine

Sea salt and black pepper

Directions:

1. Add all of the chicken ingredients to a large bowl and toss to combine.
2. In a second small bowl, whisk together the marinade ingredients and pour over the chicken and apricot mixture. Cover with plastic wrap and chill overnight.
3. One hour before you wish to cook, remove the chicken from the refrigerator and allow to stand at room temperature.
4. Preheat the main oven to 375 degrees F.
5. Transfer the chicken and marinade to a baking dish, along with the wine ingredients and place in the oven. Bake for 50-55 minutes, basting the chicken with the juices every 15 minutes, until the chicken is cooked through.

Freestyle SmartPoints Per Serving: 9

(Calories 270 | Total Fats 10g | Net Carbs: 3g | Protein 30g | Fiber: 4g)

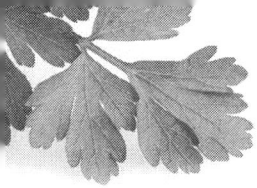

Baked Pesto Chicken

(Prep Time: 10 MIN | Cook Time: 25 MIN | Serves: 4)

Ingredients:

For cooking:
Nonstick spray

For chicken:
1 pound skinless, boneless chicken breasts (butterflied)

Sea salt and black pepper

¼ cup pesto

1 cup cherry tomatoes (halved)

½ cup low-fat mozzarella cheese (grated)

Directions:

1. Preheat the main oven to 400 degrees F. Cover a baking sheet with kitchen foil and spritz with nonstick spray.
2. Season each butterflied chicken breast with sea salt and black pepper and spread with pesto.
3. Arrange on the baking sheet along with the tomatoes, and place in the oven for 15-17 minutes until cooked.
4. Remove and sprinkle with the grated cheese, return to the oven and cook for 5-6 minutes until the cheese melts.

Freestyle SmartPoints Per Serving: 3

(Calories 220 | Total Fats 10g | Net Carbs: 3g | Protein 28g | Fiber: 1g)

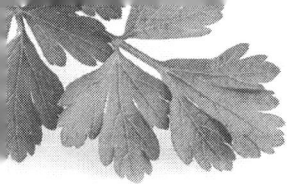

Cheddar, Turkey, and Broccoli Potato Skins

(Prep Time: 15 MIN | Cook Time: 1 HOUR 25 MIN | Serves: 10)

Ingredients:

For cooking:
Nonstick spray

For potatoes:
5 (10 ounce) russet potatoes

Sea salt

1½ cups cooked, chopped turkey breast

2 cups cooked, chopped broccoli

For filling:
1¼ cups low-fat Cheddar cheese (shredded)

¼ cup low-fat sour cream

¼ cup skim milk

2 tbsp onion flakes

2½ tsp seasoned salt

1 tsp powdered garlic

1½ cups cooked, chopped turkey breast

2 cups cooked, chopped broccoli

Directions:

1. Preheat the main oven to 400 degrees F.
2. Spritz a baking sheet with nonstick spray. Arrange the potatoes on the sheet, spritz with more nonstick spray and season with sea salt.
3. Place in the oven and bake for approximately 50 minutes, until done.
4. Take the cooked potatoes out of the oven and turn the temperature down to 350 degrees F.
5. Allow the potatoes to cool a little before slicing in half. Scoop the flesh from the potato halves and add to a large bowl, along with all of the other filling ingredients (excluding the turkey and broccoli). Mash until well combined.
6. Add the cooked turkey and broccoli and stir well.
7. Spoon the filling mixture equally into the empty potato halves and rearrange on the baking tray.
8. Place in the oven and bake for 15-18 minutes, until the filling is heated through. Serve hot.

Freestyle SmartPoints Per Serving: 5

(Calories 235 | Total Fats 1g | Net Carbs: 43g | Protein 12g | Fiber: 3g)

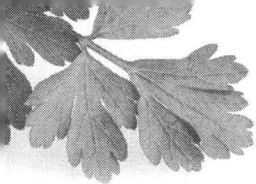

Chicken in Herby Wine and Mushroom Sauce

(Prep Time: 10 MIN | Cook Time: 35 MIN | Serves: 6)

Ingredients:

For cooking:

½ tbsp olive oil

For chicken:

1½ pounds boneless, skinless
chicken thighs

1 tbsp olive oil

1 tsp basil

1 tsp oregano

1 tsp thyme

1 tsp parsley

Sea salt and black pepper

For sauce:

4 cloves garlic (peeled,
minced)

8 ounces mushrooms (sliced)

½ cup dry red wine

1 cup skim milk

1 tbsp cornstarch mixed with 1
tbsp water

¼ cup Parmesan cheese
(shredded)

2 tbsp fresh parsley (roughly
chopped)

Directions:

1. Preheat the main oven to 400 degrees F.
2. Add all of the chicken ingredients to a large bowl and toss well to coat.
3. Add the coated chicken to a skillet over moderately high heat and fry in the olive oil for 3 minutes on each side until crispy.
4. Transfer the skillet and chicken to the oven and cook for just over 20 minutes, until cooked through.
5. Set the chicken to one side and return the skillet to the stovetop and cook the garlic over moderately high heat for 60 seconds, before adding the mushrooms and a pinch more salt.
6. Pour in the wine and cook until the liquid reduces by half. Add the milk, stir, and bring to a simmer stirring often.
7. Add the cornstarch mixture and stir the sauce very well.
8. Sprinkle with the Parmesan and wait for it to melt before returning the chicken to the skillet. Simmer for a couple more minutes, before garnishing with parsley and serving.

Freestyle SmartPoints Per Serving: 6

(Calories 295 | Total Fats 11g | Net Carbs: 5.5g | Protein 36g | Fiber: 0.5g)

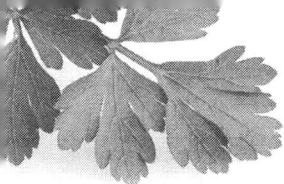

Chicken Sausages with Spicy Pineapple Salsa

(Prep Time: 10 MIN | Cook Time: 10 MIN | Serves: 4)

Ingredients:

For pineapple salsa:

⅛ cup fresh cilantro (finely chopped)

1 cup fresh pineapple (peeled and diced)

½ cup red bell pepper (deseeded and diced)

⅛ cup red onion (peeled and diced)

Juice of 1 medium lime

¼ tsp pepper

¼ tsp cumin

½ jalapeno (deseeded and diced)

¼ tsp sea salt

For sausages:

4 cooked chicken sausages

Sea salt and black pepper

Directions:

1. Add all of the salsa ingredients to a medium bowl and stir to combine.
2. Season the sausages with sea salt and black pepper before grilling for several minutes, until heated through.
3. Serve the hot sausages in your favorite Weight Watcher's friendly bun and top with plenty of spicy salsa.

Freestyle SmartPoints Per Serving: 4

(Calories 175 | Total Fats 5g | Net Carbs: 10g | Protein 16g | Fiber: 2g)

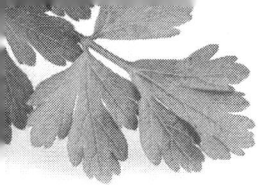

Fig and Honey Chicken with Saffron

(Prep Time: 10 MIN | Cook Time: 45 MIN | Serves: 6)

Ingredients:

For cooking:
Nonstick spray

For chicken:
1 yellow onion (peeled, thinly sliced)

2 pounds boneless, skinless chicken breasts fillets

⅓ cup organic honey

10 ounces fresh figs (cut into quarters)

For paste:
½ tsp saffron

1 tbsp olive oil

1 tsp coriander

Sea salt and black pepper

1 tsp paprika

Directions:

1. Spritz a Dutch oven with nonstick spray and place over moderately high heat.
2. Add the onions and fry for several minutes, until soft.
3. In the meantime, combine the paste ingredients in a small bowl.
4. Rub the paste into the chicken fillets and arrange in the Dutch oven.
5. Drizzle over the organic honey and reduce the heat to moderate. Cover with a lid and cook for approximately half an hour, until cooked through.
6. Approximately 15 minutes, before the chicken is cooked, add the quartered figs.
7. Remember to baste the chicken with the juices regularly to keep it moist.

Freestyle SmartPoints Per Serving: 6

(Calories 275 | Total Fats 4g | Net Carbs: 22.5g | Protein 32g | Fiber: 1.5g)

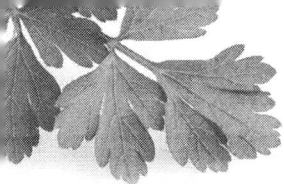

Tikka Masala

(Prep Time: 15 MIN | Cook Time: 4 HOUR | Serves: 4)

Ingredients:

For cooking:
Nonstick spray

For chicken and rice:
8 ounces boneless, skinless chicken breast
(chopped)
1 cup brown rice

For sauce:
1 yellow onion (peeled and sliced)
Juice of 1 medium lime
4 cloves garlic (peeled, minced)
1 tsp allspice
1 tsp kosher salt
½ cup fat-free plain Greek yogurt
28 ounces canned chopped tomatoes
2 jalapenos (deseeded, finely chopped)
1 tbsp fresh grated ginger
1 tbsp garam masala
½ tsp black pepper
1 tbsp cumin
1 tsp paprika
¼ cup fresh cilantro (roughly chopped)

Directions:

1. Spritz a crockpot with nonstick spray and add all of the sauce ingredients. Stir well to combine.
2. Add the chopped chicken and stir again. Cover and cook for 4 hours on high heat.
3. When the Tikka Masala is almost finished cooking, prepare the rice according to packet directions.
4. Serve the chicken Tikka Masala over the cooked rice and garnish with fresh cilantro.

Freestyle SmartPoints Per Serving: 7

(Calories 295 | Total Fats 2g | Net Carbs: 40g | Protein 25g | Fiber: 5g)

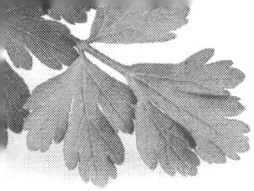

Black Pepper and Lemon Breaded Chicken

(Prep Time: 15 MIN | Cook Time: 20 MIN | Serves: 4)

Ingredients:

For cooking:
Nonstick spray

For chicken:
⅓ cup panko breadcrumbs

⅓ cup Parmesan cheese (grated)

2 medium eggs (beaten)

1⅓ pounds skinless, boneless chicken cutlets

3 cups green beans

2 tsp virgin olive oil

Sea salt and black pepper

Seasoning:
1 tsp lemon pepper

½ tsp garlic powder

Salt and black pepper

Directions:

1. Preheat the main oven to 425 degrees F. Spritz a baking sheet with nonstick spray.
2. In a bowl, combine the breadcrumbs with the Parmesan cheese, and seasonings.
3. Add the beaten egg to a shallow bowl.
4. Dip one side of the chicken in the beaten egg and then into the breadcrumb-Parmesan mixture. Place the chicken on the prepared baking sheet with the breaded side facing upwards.
5. Toss the green beans with the virgin oil and season with salt and black pepper. Spread the beans evenly out on the prepared baking sheet around the breaded chicken.
6. Cook in the preheated oven for 15 minutes, until the chicken's juices run clear and the meat is tender.

Freestyle Smart Points Per Serving: 3

(Calories 299 | Total Fats 10g | Net Carbs: 8g | Protein 43g | Fiber: 2g)

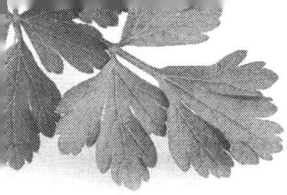

Buffalo Chicken Wings

(Prep Time: 10 MIN | Cook Time: 1 HOUR 5 MIN | Serves: 8)

Ingredients:

For cooking:
Nonstick spray

For bake:
2 pounds chicken wings
(frozen)
2 tbsp butter
4 tbsp buffalo sauce

Directions:

1. Add the chicken wings to a microwave-safe bowl. Pour in sufficient water to cover halfway up the wings. On a high setting, microwave for 10 minutes. Remove from the microwave and stir. Return to the microwave and again, on high, microwave for 10 minutes.

2. Preheat the main oven to 450 degrees F.

3. Using kitchen tongs remove the chicken wings from the water and pat dry using kitchen paper towel.

4. Using aluminum foil, cover a baking tray and generously mist with nonstick cooking spray.

5. In an even, single layer arrange the wings on the baking tray and bake in the preheated oven for 40 minutes. Flip the chicken wings over and bake for a further 10 minutes.

6. As the chicken wings approach the end of the cooking process, melt the butter in the baking tray, add the buffalo sauce and stir to combine.

7. Allow the wings to cool for several minutes, toss with the buffalo sauce and enjoy.

Freestyle Smart Points Per Serving: 7

(Calories 277 | Total Fats 21g | Net Carbs: 0g | Protein 21g | Fiber: 0g)

Ginger Soy Chicken with Fruity Mango Salsa

(Prep Time: 4 HOUR 10MIN | Cook Time: 10 MIN | Serves: 4)

Ingredients:

For cooking:

Nonstick spray

For salsa:

1 ripe, medium mango (peeled, pitted, diced)

¼ cup red onion (peeled, finely chopped)

¼ cup fresh cilantro (roughly chopped)

Juice of 1 medium lime

Salt and black pepper

For marinated chicken:

1⅓ pounds skinless, boneless chicken breast

¼ cup low-sodium soy sauce

2 tbsp freshly squeezed orange juice

1 tbsp fresh ginger (peeled, minced)

2 cloves garlic (peeled, minced)

1 tbsp sesame oil

½ tsp black pepper

Directions:

1. Cut the chicken breasts into tenders and add to a Ziploc bag along with the remaining marinating ingredients. Transfer to the refrigerator for 4 hours.
2. When you are ready to grill, take the chicken out of the Ziploc bag, allowing any excess marinade to drip off. Transfer the chicken to a hot grill, and cook until the chicken's juices run clear, this will take around 3-5 minutes, each side.
3. Next prepare the salsa by combining all of the ingredients in a small bowl.
4. Spoon the salsa over the cooked chicken and serve.

Freestyle Smart Points Per Serving: 2

(Calories 252 | Total Fats 6g | Net Carbs: 16g | Protein 34g | Fiber: 2g)

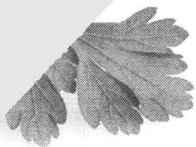

Sweet Pineapple BBQ Chicken

(Prep Time: 8 HOUR 15 MIN | Cook Time: 15 MIN | Serves: 4)

Ingredients:

For cooking:

Nonstick spray

For marinating sauce:

½ cup BBQ sauce

¼ cup fresh pineapple juice

2 tbsp soy sauce

1 clove garlic (minced)

1 tsp Asian hot sauce

1 tsp ginger (minced)

For chicken:

1⅓ pounds skinless, boneless chicken breast

2 cups fresh pineapple (peeled, cored, sliced)

Directions:

1. Combine all of the ingredients for marinating in a large bowl and add the chicken, cover, and chill overnight.

2. When you are ready to cook, take the chicken out of the marinade and allow any excess to drip off. Lightly mist the slices of pineapple with nonstick spray. Grill the pineapple along with the chicken for 5 minutes each side or until sufficiently cooked. Cooking time will vary depending on the thickness of the chicken.

3. In the meantime, add the excess marinade to a small pan. Bring to boil, and cook until slightly reduced, for approximately 5 minutes. Drizzle the marinade over the chicken and pineapple and serve.

Freestyle Smart Points Per Serving: 4

(Calories 270 | Total Fats 2g | Net Carbs: 23g | Protein 33g | Fiber: 2g)

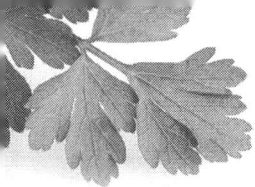

Take-Out Style Kung Pao Chicken

(Prep Time: 10 MIN | Cook Time: 15 MIN | Serves: 4)

Ingredients:

For cooking:
4 tsp sesame oil

For chicken:
1⅓ pounds skinless, boneless chicken breast (chopped)

2 cloves garlic (peeled, minced)

1 tsp ginger (peeled, minced)

2 celery ribs (chopped)

1 red pepper (seeded, chopped)

2 green scallions (chopped)

For sauce:
2 tbsp low sodium soy sauce

1 ½ tsp Sriracha

1 tbsp runny honey

½ tsp black pepper

¼ cup peanuts (chopped)

Directions:

1. Add half of the sesame oil to a frying pan. Add the chopped chicken followed by the garlic and ginger. Cook until just cooked through, for between 5-7 minutes.
2. Add the remaining oil to the frying pan along with the celery and red pepper; cook until crisp yet tender, 5-7 minutes.
3. In the meantime, combine the sauce ingredients in a small bowl.
4. Return the chicken to the pan and pour over the sauce. Cook for a couple of minutes; until the sauce thickens.
5. Take the pan off the heat and put to one side to rest for 2-3 minutes.
6. Garnish with scallions.

Freestyle Smart Points Per Serving: 3

(Calories 303 | Total Fats 11g | Net Carbs: 9g | Protein 36g | Fiber: 2g)

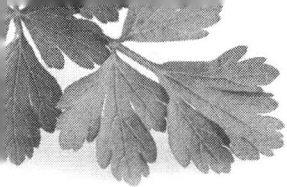

Turkey BBQ Meatloaves

(Prep Time: 15 MIN | Cook Time: 30 MIN | Serves: 5)

Ingredients:

For cooking:

Nonstick spray

1¼ tsp virgin olive oil

For bake:

½ onion (peeled, minced)

2 cloves garlic (peeled, minced)

1¾ pounds lean ground turkey (99% fat-free)

5 tbsp tomato ketchup

1 tbsp mustard

1 tbsp Worcestershire sauce

2½ tsp grill seasoning

1 medium egg (beaten)

Salt (to season)

5 tbsp BBQ sauce (no added sugar)

Directions:

1. Preheat the main oven to 350 degrees F. Spritz a 10-hole muffin tin with nonstick spray.
2. In a frying pan or skillet, sauté the onion and garlic in the olive oil until fork tender, this will take around 4-6 minutes.
3. Combine the cooked onions and garlic with the turkey, ketchup, mustard, Worcestershire sauce, seasoning, and egg. Taste and season with salt if necessary.
4. Evenly divide the meatloaf mixture between the 10 muffin tin holes. Using a pastry brush, lightly glaze the top of each mini meatloaf with BBQ sauce.
5. Bake in the preheated oven for 20-25 minutes.

Freestyle Smart Points Per Serving: 2

(Calories 243 | Total Fats 5g | Net Carbs: 12g | Protein 38g | Fiber: 0g)

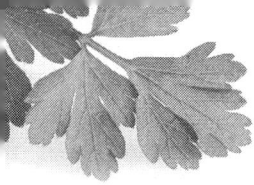

Turkey Bolognese with Zucchini Noodles

(Prep Time: 10 MIN | Cook Time: 25 MIN | Serves: 4)

Ingredients:

For cooking:
2 tbsp virgin olive oil

For bolognese:
1 celery stalk (diced)

1 carrot (diced)

½ sweet onion (peeled, diced)

1⅓ pounds lean ground turkey (93% fat-free)

20 ounces Italian canned, crushed tomatoes

1 tbsp tomato paste

4 zucchini

⅓ cup fresh basil (chopped)

Seasoning:
3 garlic cloves (peeled, minced)

1 tsp red pepper flakes

Sea salt and black pepper (to season)

½ tbsp oregano

Directions:

1. Add the olive oil to a large frying pan over moderate heat.
2. Add the celery followed by the carrots and onion and cook for between 4-5 minutes.
3. Next, add the turkey and, using the back of a wooden spoon, gently break up the meat and cook until it is no longer pink. Add the seasoning and stir.
4. Pour in the tomatoes and tomato paste. Bring to simmer and cover with a tight-fitting lid. Allow to simmer for a minimum of 15 minutes.
5. In the meantime, using a vegetable spiralizer or peeler, cut the zucchini into thin ribbons/noodles.
6. Add the zucchini noodles to the sauce and cook until fork tender, this will take 3-5 minutes.
7. Add the fresh basil, stir to combine and season to taste.

Freestyle Smart Points Per Serving: 7

(Calories 417 | Total Fats 21g | Net Carbs: 19g | Protein 36g | Fiber: 8g)

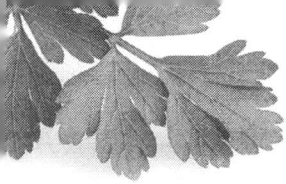

Cordon Bleu Skillet Chicken

(Prep Time: 15 MIN | Cook Time: 15 MIN | Serves: 4)

Ingredients:

For cooking:

1½ tsp olive oil

½ tsp salted butter

For chicken:

4 (4 ounce) skinless, boneless chicken cutlets

½ tsp sea salt

Pinch black pepper

¼ cup all-purpose flour

4 (¾ ounce slices) reduced-salt deli ham

4 (¾ ounce slices) low-fat Swiss cheese

Fresh parsley (chopped, for garnish)

For sauce:

⅔ cup fat-free chicken stock

1 tbsp freshly squeezed lemon juice

½ tbsp Dijon mustard

1 tsp all-purpose flour

Directions:

1. Season each chicken cutlet with sea salt and black pepper.
2. Add the flour to a wide dish. Dip each cutlet in the flour to coat both sides, shake off any excess and set aside for a moment.
3. Whisk together the sauce ingredients and set to one side.
4. Melt the oil and butter in a 12" skillet over moderately high heat. Add the floured chicken cutlets and sauté for 2 minutes on both sides. Transfer the semi-cooked chicken to a plate.
5. Add the set-aside sauce mixture to the skillet and scraping up any brown bits, bring the sauce to simmer for 2-3 minutes until it reduces a little.
6. Place the chicken back in the skillet and arrange one slice of ham and one slice of cheese on top of each piece.
7. Cover the skillet with a lid and cook at a moderately low simmer for 3-4 minutes until the cheese has melted.
8. Divide the chicken between four plates and spoon a little of the remaining sauce over each portion.

Freestyle Smart Points Per Serving: 5

(Calories 260 | Total Fats 10g | Net Carbs: 6g | Protein 37g | Fiber: 0g)

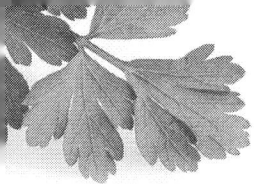

Feta and Butternut Squash Turkey Skillet

(Prep Time: 10 MIN | Cook Time: 20 MIN | Serves: 4)

Ingredients:

For cooking:

1 tbsp olive oil

For turkey:

1 pound 99% lean ground turkey
1 red bell pepper (seeded, diced)
½ yellow onion (peeled, minced)
2 cloves garlic (peeled, minced)
1 cup canned chopped tomatoes
2 cups butternut squash (peeled, seeded, chopped)
1 cup low-fat feta cheese (crumbled)

Seasoning:

Sea salt and black pepper
1 tsp Italian seasoning mix
1 tsp powdered garlic
¼ tsp crushed red pepper flakes

Directions:

1. To a large skillet, add the oil and place over moderately high heat. Add the turkey and sauté for several minutes; use a wooden spoon to break up the turkey as it cooks.
2. Add the red bell pepper, onion, and garlic, cook for another 5-6 minutes until the vegetables have softened.
3. Add the chopped tomatoes, chopped squash, and seasoning, stir well. Cover with a lid and cook for several minutes.
4. Add the feta cheese and recover for 2-3 minutes more until the cheese melts.
5. Serve.

Freestyle Smart Points Per Serving: 3

(Calories 280 | Total Fats 10g | Net Carbs: 12g | Protein 35g | Fiber: 3g)

INSTANT POT POULTRY DISHES

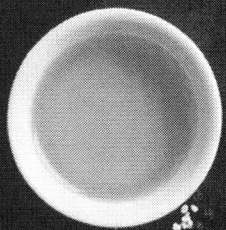

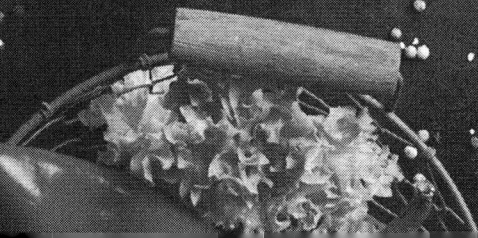

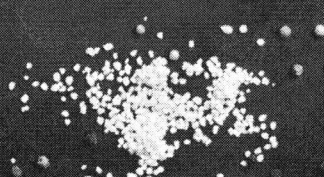

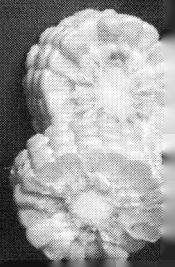

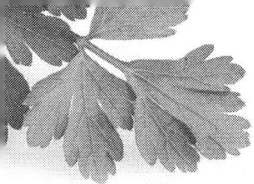

Salsa Verde Chicken

(Prep Time: 15 MIN | Cook Time: 18 MIN | Serves: 0)

Ingredients:

For cooking:

Nonstick spray

For chicken:

2 lbs chicken fillets, thinly sliced

½ cup green peas, frozen

1 medium-sized onion, chopped

½ tsp salt

¼ tsp black pepper, ground

¼ tsp dried thyme, ground

For salsa verde sauce:

4 tsp extra virgin olive oil

2 tsp red wine vinegar

½ tsp garlic powder

2 tbsp fresh basil, finely chopped

2 tbsp fresh parsley, final chopped

1 tbsp fresh mint, finely chopped

2 tsp capers, reduced sodium

2 anchovies, reduced sodium

1 tsp Dijon mustard

½ tsp sea salt

½ tsp black pepper, ground

Directions:

1. In a small mixing bowl, combine all salsa verde ingredients. Mix until well combined and set aside.
2. Rinse the fillets under running water. Pat dry with a kitchen paper and sprinkle with some salt, pepper and thyme. Set aside. Plug in the Instant Pot and grease the stainless steel insert with some cooking spray. Press the Sauté button and heat up the pot. Add onions and cook for 3-4 minutes, or until the onions are translucent. Add chicken fillets and cook for 3-4 minutes on each side. Remove from the pot.
3. Add beans and pour 1 cup of water. Securely lock the lid and adjust the steam release handle. Press the Manual button and set the timer for 8 minutes on High pressure.
4. When done, perform a quick pressure release and open the pot.
5. Serve chicken with peas and drizzle with some salsa verde sauce.
6. Enjoy!

Freestyle SmartPoints Per Serving: 5

(Calories 261 | Total Fats 11.3g | Net Carbs: 2.1g | Protein 35.1g | Fiber: 0.9g)

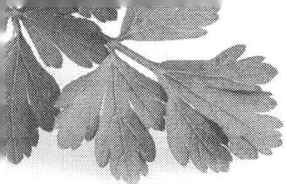

Chicken Broccoli Linguine

(Prep Time: 20 MIN | Cook Time: 13 MIN | Serves: 5)

Ingredients:

For cooking:

2 tsp olive oil

For chicken broccoli:

1 lb chicken fillets, cut into bite-sized pieces

1 cup broccoli, chopped into florets

1 tsp soy sauce, reduced sodium

2 tbsp chicken broth, reduced sodium

½ tsp garlic powder

½ tsp onion powder

½ tsp dried oregano, ground

¼ tsp sea salt

¼ tsp smoked paprika

For linguine pasta:

8 oz linguine pasta

1 tsp butter

¼ tsp salt

¼ tsp dried thyme

Directions:

1. Combine soy sauce, chicken broth, garlic powder, onion powder, oregano, salt, and smoked paprika in a small mixing bowl.

2. Grease the stainless steel insert of your Instant Pot with olive oil. Press Sauté button and heat up. Add chicken and broccoli and cook for 5 minutes, stirring occasionally. Pour in the previously prepared sauce and give it a good stir. Cook for 2 more minutes. Remove to a large bowl and cover with a lid.

3. Now, pour 1 ½ cup of water in the inner pot. Add pasta and sprinkle with some salt and thyme. Securely lock the lid and set the steam release handle by moving the valve to the Sealing position. Press the Manual button and set the timer for 4 minutes. Cook on High pressure.

4. When done, perform a quick pressure release and open the pot. Drain the pasta and remove the liquid.

5. Add the butter to the pot. Using a wooden spatula, stir until melts over a Sauté mode. Return the pasta to the pot and cook for 2 minutes, stirring constantly.

6. Transfer the pasta to a serving plate and top with chicken. Garnish with some basil leaves and serve immediately.

Freestyle SmartPoints Per Serving: 4

(Calories 199 | Total Fats 8.7g | Net Carbs: 1.3g | Protein 27.1g | Fiber: 0.6g)

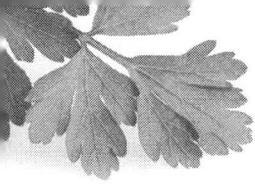

Mozzarella Tomato Turkey

(Prep Time: 10 MIN | Cook Time: 10 MIN | Serves: 4)

Ingredients:

For cooking:

Nonstick cooking spray

For turkey:

1 lb turkey breasts, cut into bite-sized pieces
½ tsp dried thyme, ground
¼ tsp dried rosemary, ground
1 tsp tomato paste

For Mozzarella tomato:

1 cup Roma tomatoes, diced
¼ cup Mozzarella cheese
1 tsp dry sherry
2 tsp fresh basil, finely chopped
¼ tsp sea salt

Directions:

1. Rinse the fillets under running water and pat dry with a kitchen paper. Cut into bite-sized pieces and place in a bowl. Add tomato paste, thyme, rosemary, salt, and pepper. Using your hands, mix to coat all. Set aside.

2. Plug in the Instant Pot and spray the stainless steel insert with some nonstick cooking spray. Press the Sauté button and add turkey chops. Cook for 5 minutes, stirring occasionally.

3. Add diced tomatoes, mozzarella, dry sherry, basil, and salt. Stir well and bring it to a boil. Simmer for 5 more minutes.

4. Turn off the pot and transfer all to a serving bowl.

5. Optionally, drizzle with some lemon juice and garnish with some fresh parsley before serving. Enjoy!

Freestyle SmartPoints Per Serving: 3

(Calories 136 | Total Fats 2.3g | Net Carbs: 5.7g | Protein 20.3g | Fiber: 1.3g)

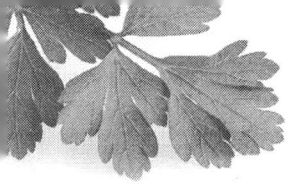

Orange Glazed Duck

(Prep Time: 15 MIN | Cook Time: 15 MIN | Serves: 4)

Ingredients:

For cooking:

1 cup chicken stock, reduced sodium

2 tsp dry sherry

For orange sauce:

1 large orange, freshly juiced

1 tsp butter, melted

1 tsp red wine vinegar

1 tsp all-purpose flour

1 tsp sugar

For duck:

1 lb duck breasts, skinless and boneless

1 small red onion, chopped

¼ cup baby carrot, sliced

1 tbsp fresh parsley, finely chopped

Seasoning:

1 tsp fresh thyme, finely chopped

1 tsp fresh rosemary, finely chopped

½ tsp cumin, ground

Salt

Black pepper

Directions:

1. Plug in the Instant Pot and pour the chicken stock and dry sherry in the stainless steel insert. Add meat and vegetables. Sprinkle with thyme, rosemary, cumin, salt, and pepper. Stir well and pour ½ cup of water in.
2. Securely lock the lid and adjust the steam release handle by turning the valve to the Sealing position. Press the Manual button and set the timer for 8 minutes. Cook on High pressure.
3. Meanwhile, combine all sauce ingredients in a small saucepan over medium-high heat. Stir well and bring it to a boil. Remove from the heat and set aside.
4. When you hear the cooker's end signal, perform a quick pressure release and open the pot.
5. Stir in the orange sauce and press the Sauté button. Cook for 2 more minutes and turn off the pot.
6. Transfer to a serving dish and sprinkle with some finely chopped parsley.

Freestyle SmartPoints Per Serving: 3

(Calories 160 | Total Fats 4.7g | Net Carbs: 1.6g | Protein 25.3g | Fiber: 0.4g)

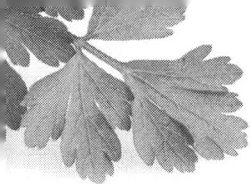

Spicy Turkey Risotto

(Prep Time: 10 MIN | Cook Time: 10 MIN | Serves: 6)

Ingredients:

For cooking:

Nonstick cooking spray

For turkey risotto:

8 oz turkey breasts, skinless, boneless and cut into bite-sized pieces

1 ½ cup brown rice

3 large egg whites

¼ cup spring onions, finely chopped

1 small carrot, cut into small cubes

1 tbsp soy sauce, reduced sodium

Seasoning:

½ tsp garlic powder

½ tsp turmeric powder

1 tsp chili powder

Salt

Black pepper

Directions:

1. Plug in the Instant Pot and grease the stainless steel insert with some cooking spray. Press the Sauté button and add turkey. Sprinkle with some garlic powder, salt, and pepper. Cook for 5 minutes, or until golden brown.

2. Remove the turkey from the pot and add egg whites. Cook for 2 minutes and then transfer to a bowl with turkey. Cover with a lid and set aside.

3. Now, add rice and carrots to the pot. Sprinkle with turmeric powder, chili powder, and some salt to taste. Stir well and pour in 2 cups of water. Press the Rice mode and set the timer for 7 minutes. Cook on High pressure.

4. When done perform a quick pressure release and open the pot. Stir in the soy sauce and green onions. Press the Sauté button and cook for another 2 minutes.

5. Stir in the egg whites and turn off the pot.

6. Transfer all to a bowl with turkey and give it a good stir to combine. Enjoy!

Freestyle SmartPoints Per Serving: 6

(Calories 226 | Total Fats 1.9g | Net Carbs: 37.1g | Protein 12.1g | Fiber: 2.1g)

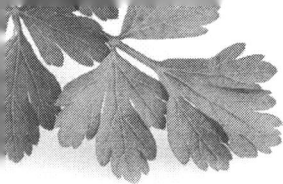

Turkey in Mushroom Gravy

(Prep Time: 10 MIN | Cook Time: 18 MIN | Serves: 6)

Ingredients:

For cooking:
Nonstick cooking spray

For turkey:
1 lb turkey breasts, skinless, boneless, and cut into bite-sized pieces

1 small red onion, sliced

1 medium-sized red bell pepper, chopped

1 garlic clove, minced

For mushroom gravy:
1 cup button mushrooms, sliced

¼ cup skim milk

1 tbsp all-purpose flour

1 tsp soy sauce, reduced sodium

½ tsp smoked paprika, ground

½ tsp black pepper, ground

Directions:

1. Plug in the Instant Pot and grease the stainless steel insert with some nonstick cooking spray. Add red pepper, onion, and garlic. Stir-fry for 3-4 minutes, or until the onions translucent. Remove the vegetables from the pot to a bowl and cover with a lid. Set aside.

2. Now, add turkey breasts and cook for 4 minutes on each side, or until golden brown. Remove from the pot and set aside, covered.

3. Place the mushrooms in the pot and pour in 1 cup of water. Press the Manual button and set the timer for 4 minutes. Cook on High pressure.

4. When done, perform a quick pressure release and open the pot. Stir in the milk, soy sauce, all-purpose flour, smoked paprika, and pepper. Press the Sauté button and simmer for 3-4 minutes, or until the gravy thickens.

5. Serve turkey breasts with bell pepper and onions. Top with mushroom gravy and serve immediately. Enjoy!

Freestyle SmartPoints Per Serving: 2

(Calories 103 | Total Fats 1.4g | Net Carbs: 6.9g | Protein 14.2g | Fiber: 1.2g)

SEAFOOD

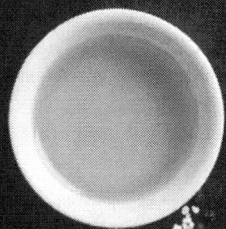
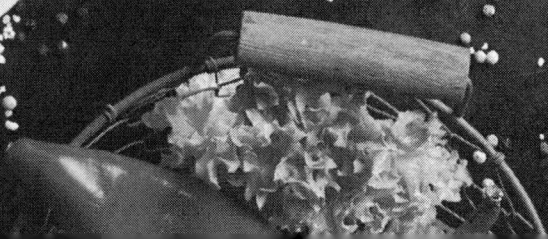
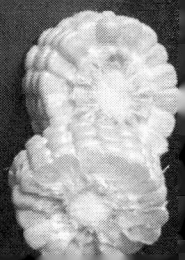

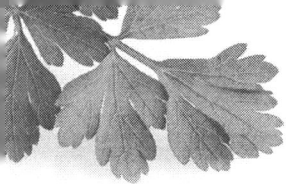

Coconut Lime Baked Mahi Mahi

(Prep Time: 20 MIN | Cook Time: 35 MIN | Serves: 4)

Ingredients:

For cooking:

Nonstick spray

For fish:

1½ pounds mahi-mahi (cut into 6)

1 red bell pepper (thinly sliced)

1 medium carrot (thinly sliced)

1 red onion (peeled, thinly sliced)

1 medium lime (seeded, sliced into 8 rings)

For marinade:

1 (13½ ounce) can light coconut milk

Freshly squeezed juice of 1 lime

1 tbsp fish sauce

1 jalapeno pepper (seeded, minced)

2 tbsp fresh ginger (peeled, sliced)

3 cloves garlic (peeled, minced)

½ cup cilantro (chopped)

½ cup Thai basil (chopped)

Directions:

1. In a bowl, combine the marinade ingredients.
2. Add the mahi-mahi to the marinade, flip over to coat, cover and transfer to the fridge for 30-60 minutes.
3. Take the fish out of the marinade and set the marinade to one side.
4. Preheat the main oven to 425 degrees F. Spritz a baking tray with nonstick spray. Toss the bell pepper, carrot, and onion evenly in the marinade. When coated, arrange the vegetables on the tray and roast for 15 minutes, or until browned.
5. Reduce the oven temperature to 325 degrees F.
6. Cut 4 large sheets of foil. In the middle of each, arrange a ¼ of the vegetables, top with one portion of fish, 1 tbsp marinade and 1 lime ring. Fold the aluminum foil around the mahi-mahi and vegetables to make a parcel. Transfer to the baking tray and cook for between 18-20 minutes.
7. Pour the remaining marinade into a pan and set over moderately high heat. Allow the marinade to reduce, while continually whisking until the sauce has thickened.
8. Remove the parcels and place each one on a dinner plate.
9. Serve each portion of fish with the sauce.

Freestyle SmartPoints Per Serving: 4

(Calories 173 | Total Fats 5g | Net Carbs: 3g | Protein 22g | Fiber: 2g)

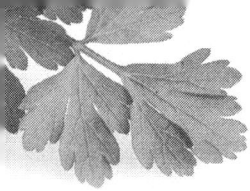

Crab Cakes with Homemade Chipotle Sauce

(Prep Time: 40 MIN | Cook Time: 25 MIN | Serves: 8)

Ingredients:

For cooking:

Nonstick cooking spray

For chipotle sauce:

½ cup jarred roasted red bell peppers (drained)

¼ cup fat-free Greek yogurt

1 tbsp mayonnaise

Juice of ½ a medium lime

2 tsp chipotle pepper seasoning

1 clove garlic (peeled)

Sea salt and black pepper

For crab cakes:

1 pound crab meat

⅔ cup Panko breadcrumbs

¼ cup non-fat Greek yogurt

Juice of ½ a medium lime

1 medium egg

1 medium egg white

4 scallions

¼ cup fresh cilantro (finely chopped)

½ large, red bell pepper (finely chopped)

Sea salt and black pepper

Directions:

1. Preheat the main oven to 400 degrees F. Spritz a large baking sheet with nonstick spray.
2. In a bowl, combine all of the crab cake ingredients. Cover the bowl and allow to chill in the fridge for 30 minutes.
3. Form the mixture into 16 patties and arrange them on the cookie sheet. Bake in the oven for 12 minutes on each side.
4. In the meantime, combine all of the sauce ingredients in a small bowl.
5. Drizzle the sauce over the 16 crab cakes and serve.

Freestyle SmartPoints Per Serving: 3

(Calories 103 | Total Fats 2.5g | Net Carbs: 8g | Protein 12g | Fiber: 0g)

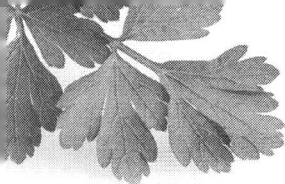

Ginger and Honey Glazed Cod

(Prep Time: 5 MIN | Cook Time: 5 MIN | Serves: 4)

Ingredients:

For cooking:
Nonstick spray

For sauce:
3 tbsp honey

3 tbsp low-salt soy sauce

2 tbsp freshly squeezed lemon juice

1 tsp sesame oil

1 tsp ginger (peeled, grated)

For the fish:
4 cod fillets

Directions:

1. Combine all of the sauce ingredients in a small bowl.
2. Spritz a baking sheet with nonstick spray.
3. Arrange the cod fillets on the prepared sheet. Divide the sauce between the 4 fillets.
4. Grill, until the fish flakes easily when using a fork; this will take between 3-5 minutes.

Freestyle SmartPoints Per Serving: 4

(Calories 172 | Total Fats 2g | Net Carbs: 3g | Protein 23.8g | Fiber: 12g)

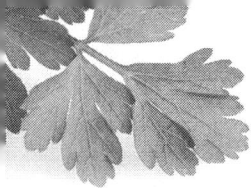

Pan-Seared Tuna

(Prep Time: 10 MIN | Cook Time: 5 MIN | Serves: 4)

Ingredients:

For cooking:
Nonstick spray

For marinade:
1 tbsp sesame oil
⅓ cup reduced sodium soy sauce
2 garlic cloves (peeled, minced)
Juice of 1 medium lime
1 tsp fresh ginger (grated)

For fish:
4 (4 ounce) Ahi tuna steaks
1 green onion (chopped, to serve)

Directions:

1. Add all of the marinade ingredients to a bowl and stir to combine.
2. Add the tuna steaks to the marinade. Cover the bowl and transfer to the fridge for at least 60 minutes.
3. Spritz a large, frying pan with nonstick spray and set over moderately high heat.
4. As soon as the pan is sufficiently hot, sear the tuna for 1½-2 minutes on each side, depending on your preferred level of doneness.
5. Remove the tuna from the pan and serve with green onions.

Freestyle SmartPoints Per Serving: 4

(Calories 210 | Total Fats 5g | Net Carbs: 2g | Protein 27g | Fiber: 0g)

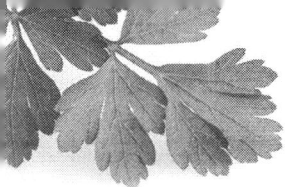

Paprika Roasted Cod

(Prep Time: 10 MIN | Cook Time: 15 MIN | Serves: 6)

Ingredients:

For cooking:
Nonstick spray

For seasoning:
1 tsp paprika
1 tsp garlic powder
1 tsp Old Bay seasoning
1 tsp thyme
Sea salt
Freshly ground black pepper

For fish:
2 pounds cod (cut into 6 fillets)
Juice of 1 medium lemon
1 tbsp olive oil

Directions:

1. Preheat the main oven to 400 degrees F. Spritz a casserole dish with nonstick spray.
2. In a bowl, combine the seasoning ingredients.
3. Arrange the fish fillets in the casserole dish, sprinkle with the juice of 1 lemon and brush with 1 tbsp of olive oil. Evenly coat the fillets with the seasoning mix.
4. Bake in the oven, until the fish flakes easily when using a fork, this will take around 12-15 minutes. Serve.

Freestyle SmartPoints Per Serving: 6

(Calories 145 | Total Fats 3g | Net Carbs: 0g | Protein 27g | Fiber: 0g)

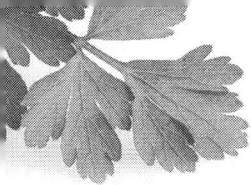

Parmesan Crusted Tilapia

(Prep Time: 5 MIN | Cook Time: 10 MIN | Serves: 8)

Ingredients:

For the crust:

½ cup Parmesan cheese (grated)

¼ cup butter (softened)

3 tbsp mayonnaise

2 tbsp freshly squeezed lemon juice

¼ tsp dried basil

¼ tsp black pepper

⅛ tsp onion powder

⅛ tsp celery salt

For the fish:

2 pounds tilapia fillets

Directions:

1. Preheat a grill. Using aluminum foil, line a baking pan and set to one side.
2. In a mixing bowl, combine the crust ingredients, mixing well to incorporate. Set to one side.
3. Arrange the fish fillets on the baking pan and broil for a few minutes. Flip over and grill for another few minutes on the other side.
4. Scatter the files with the crust mixture.
5. Broil the fish for another 2 minutes, until the fish flakes easily when using a fork, and the crust is golden brown.

Freestyle SmartPoints Per Serving: 6

(Calories 224 | Total Fats 13g | Net Carbs: 7g | Protein 25.5g | Fiber: 1g)

SEAFOOD

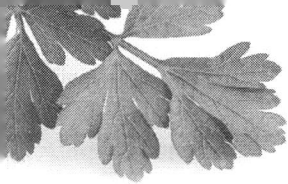

Sole in White Wine and Caper Butter

(Prep Time: 10 MIN | Cook Time: 5 MIN | Serves: 4)

Ingredients:

For cooking:
1 tbsp olive oil

For coating:
⅓ cup whole wheat flour
1 tsp sea salt
½ tsp black pepper
½ tsp paprika

For fish:
4 (4 ounce) fillets of sole fish
1 cup white wine
2 tbsp freshly squeezed lemon juice
¼ cup capers (drained)
2 tbsp light butter

Directions:

1. Combine all of the coating ingredients in a shallow bowl.
2. Using kitchen paper, pat the fish dry and dredge evenly on both sides in the coating mixture.
3. In a large frying pan, heat the oil over moderately high heat. When the oil begins to sizzle, place the fish in the frying pan and fry for a couple of minutes on each side, until golden. Remove the fish from the pan and set to one side.
4. Pour the wine into the pan, and scrape up any brown bits. Cook for 2-3 minutes, until most of the wine has reduced. Stir in the freshly squeezed lemon juice and add the capers along with the butter. Cook until the sauce bubbles and the butter is incorporated.
5. Serve with the wine sauce.

Freestyle SmartPoints Per Serving: 6

(Calories 235 | Total Fats 7.5g | Net Carbs: 8g | Protein 22g | Fiber: 1g)

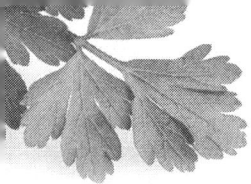

Tuna Melts

(Prep Time: 10 MIN | Cook Time: 5 MIN | Serves: 2)

Ingredients:

For cooking:

Nonstick spray

2 tbsp low-calorie butter

For tuna mayo:

1 tbsp fat-free plain Greek
yogurt

1 tbsp low-fat mayo

5 ounces canned white tuna
in water (drained)

1½ tbsp pickle relish

1 tsp Dijon mustard

For melts:

2 low-calorie whole grain
English muffins (halved,
toasted)

4 slices tomato

4 tbsp low-fat Cheddar
cheese (shredded)

Directions:

1. Preheat your oven's broiler, line a baking sheet with kitchen foil and spritz with nonstick spray.

2. Add all of the tuna mayo ingredients to a small bowl and stir to combine.

3. Arrange the toasted muffin halves on the baking tray and top each with an equal amount of tuna mayo, a tomato slice, and 1 tbsp Cheddar. Place under the broiler for a few minutes, until the cheese melts.

4. Serve straight away.

Freestyle SmartPoints Per Serving: 6

(Calories 240 | Total Fats 5g | Net Carbs: 20g | Protein 25g | Fiber: 7g)

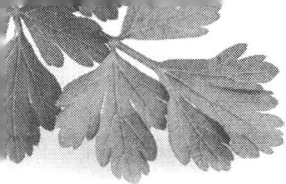

Baked Clams with Oregano

(Prep Time: 10 MIN | Cook Time: 25 MIN | Serves: 4)

Ingredients:

For cooking:

1 tbsp virgin olive oil

Nonstick spray

For breadcrumb mixture:

½ cup seasoned breadcrumbs

2 tsp oregano

1 tsp garlic powder

2 tbsp dried minced onion

2 tsp dried parsley flakes

Salt

Black pepper

For clams:

2 (6½ ounce) cans minced clams in juice

1 tbsp seasoned breadcrumbs

1 tbsp Parmesan cheese (freshly grated)

Directions:

1. Preheat the main oven to 350 degrees F.
2. In a bowl combine all ingredients for the breadcrumb mixture.
3. In a skillet, bring the olive oil to moderate heat and add the breadcrumb mixture, sauté until golden brown. Add the clams along with their juice, take off the heat and stir well.
4. Evenly divide the clam mixture between 4 ramekins. Scatter with the remaining bread crumbs and grated Parmesan. Spritz with nonstick spray.
5. Transfer to the preheated oven for 15-20 minutes, until golden.
6. Allow to cool for a few minutes before serving.

Freestyle Smart Points Per Serving: 3

(Calories 156 | Total Fats 5g | Net Carbs: 16g | Protein 11g | Fiber: 1g)

Blackened Wild Salmon with Veggie Noodles

(Prep Time: 10 MIN | Cook Time: 15 MIN | Serves: 4)

Ingredients:

For cooking:
2 tbsp olive oil

Seasoning:
2 tsp smoked paprika

½ tsp sea salt

½ tsp garlic powder

½ tsp black pepper

¼ tsp onion powder

¼ tsp dried oregano

⅛ tsp chili powder

For salmon:
1⅓ pounds skinless wild salmon fillets

2 zucchini (cut into noodles)

Salt and pepper

2 cloves garlic (peeled, minced)

1 cup cherry tomatoes

4 lemon wedges (to squeeze)

Directions:

1. In a bowl combine the seasonings.
2. Using kitchen paper towel, dry the salmon fillets. Coat the salmon on both sides with the seasoning mixture.
3. Using a spiralizer or vegetable peeler, prepare the noodles. Add the spiralized noodles to a colander and sprinkle with salt and pepper to remove a little of the moisture.
4. Over moderate heat, in a large skillet, heat half of the oil.
5. Cook the fillets for approximately 3-5 minutes each side. Remove from the skillet and set to one side, tenting with aluminum foil.
6. Add the remaining 1 tbsp of oil to the skillet together with the minced garlic and cook for 60 seconds.
7. Add the noodles along with the tomatoes and cook until al dente, for around 3-5 minutes.
8. Season to taste.
9. Arrange the salmon on top of the noodles and serve with a wedge of lemon.

Freestyle Smart Points Per Serving: 2

(Calories 331 | Total Fats 17g | Net Carbs: 7g | Protein 36g | Fiber: 3g)

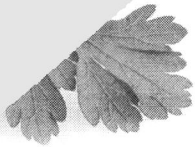

Cod and Shrimp Stew

(Prep Time: 5 MIN | Cook Time: 35 MIN | Serves: 6)

Ingredients:

For cooking:
1 tbsp virgin olive oil

For stew:
1 onion (peeled, diced)
2 cloves garlic (peeled, minced)
¼ tsp red pepper flakes
⅔ cup parsley
3 tbsp tomato paste
8 ounces bottled clam juice
14 ounces fish stock
2 tbsp butter
1½ pounds cod (sliced into 2" pieces)
1 pound raw shrimp

Seasoning:
½ tsp oregano
½ tsp basil
Salt and pepper

Directions:

1. Over moderate heat, heat the oil. Add the onion and sauté until translucent, this will take between 5-7 minutes. Add the minced garlic followed by the pepper flakes and cook for 1-2 minutes, while continually stirring. Add the parsley and cook for a couple of minutes. Add the tomato paste and cook while stirring for 60 seconds.

2. Add the tomatoes along with the clam juice and stock. Bring to simmer and add the butter and seasoning. Simmer for 12-15 minutes.

3. As soon as the broth comes to a simmer, add the cod and cook for 5 minutes.

4. Finally, add the shrimp and cook until opaque and sufficiently cooked through, this will take between 4-5 minutes.

5. Serve.

Freestyle Smart Points Per Serving: 2

(Calories 271 | Total Fats 7g | Net Carbs: 7g | Protein 42g | Fiber: 3g)

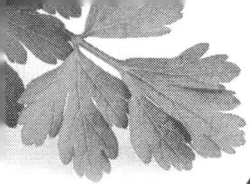

Grilled Shrimp Tostadas with Homemade Guacamole

(Prep Time: 15 MIN | Cook Time: 5 MIN | Serves: 4)

Ingredients:

For cooking:

Nonstick spray

For shrimp:

16 jumbo shrimp (shelled, deveined)

Salt

1 garlic clove (peeled, crushed)

2 tbsp store-bought salsa verde

4 tostada shells

1 (14-ounce) can fat-free refried beans

1 cup romaine lettuce (shredded)

For guacamole:

Flesh of 1 medium Hass avocado

½ plum tomato (seeded, diced)

Juice of ½ lime

2 tbsp red onion (peeled, minced)

1 small garlic clove (peeled, mashed)

½ tbsp cilantro (chopped)

Sea salt

Black pepper

Directions:

1. Add the avocado flesh to a medium bowl and mash until smooth, yet still chunky. Add the remaining guacamole ingredients to the bowl and stir to incorporate.
2. Lightly season the shrimp with salt, and coat with crushed garlic and salsa.
3. Divide the shrimp into 4 equal portions and thread onto 4 wooden skewers.
4. Light the grill on a moderate flame. Once sufficiently hot, spritz the grates with nonstick spray and grill the shrimp for between 1-2 minutes each side. Set to one side.
5. Arrange each tostada shell on a clean plate, and top each with a ¼ cup each of refried beans, lettuce and prepared guacamole.
6. Top with a shrimp skewer and serve.

Freestyle Smart Points Per Serving: 4

(Calories 262 | Total Fats 11g | Net Carbs: 14g | Protein 22g | Fiber: 6g)

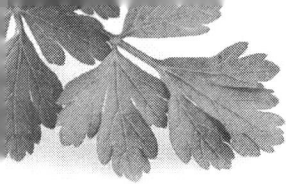

Mussels Marinara

(Prep Time: 10 MIN | Cook Time: 20 MIN | Serves: 6)

Ingredients:

For cooking:

1 tbsp virgin olive oil

For mussels:

¼ cup shallot (minced)

2 cloves garlic (peeled, thinly sliced)

1 tsp red peppercorns (crushed)

¾ cup dry white wine

1 (25¼ ounce) jar marinara sauce

3 pounds live mussels (scrubbed, de-bearded)

Sea salt

2 tbsp parsley (chopped, to garnish)

Directions:

1. Over moderately high heat, in a large pot, heat the olive oil until hot.
2. Add the shallot followed by the garlic and red pepper and cook for 60 seconds, until fragrant.
3. Pour in the wine and boil for 3 minutes, until reduced.
4. Add the marinara sauce, stir to combine and bring to simmer.
5. Add the mussels, cover with a lid and cook for between 6-8 minutes, until the mussels open. Discard any unopened mussels.
6. Lightly season with sea salt.
7. Transfer the mussels together with the sauce to a serving platter.
8. Garnish with parsley and serve.

Freestyle Smart Points Per Serving: 4

(Calories 214 | Total Fats 10g | Net Carbs: 4g | Protein 11g | Fiber: 10g)

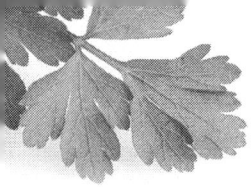

Spicy Shrimp Curry

(Prep Time: 15 MIN | Cook Time: 10 MIN | Serves: 6)

Ingredients:

For cooking:

3 tsp coconut oil

For curry:

1 pound shrimp (peeled, deveined)

½ yellow onion (peeled, finely chopped)

2 garlic cloves (peeled, minced)

1 (15-ounce) can tomato sauce

¾ cup light canned coconut milk

½ tsp kosher salt

Fresh cilantro and chili peppers (to garnish)

Seasoning:

1½ tsp ground turmeric

1 tsp ground ginger

1 tsp ground coriander

1 tsp curry powder

1 tsp ground cumin

1 tsp paprika

½ tsp chili powder

Sea salt and black pepper

Directions:

1. To a large skillet, add 2 tsp of coconut oil.
2. Add the shrimp and cook for 60 seconds on each side before removing from the skillet.
3. Add the remaining 1 tsp of oil to the skillet along with the onion. Sauté over moderate heat while occasionally stirring for 5 minutes.
4. Add the seasonings and stir to combine. Add the minced garlic. Stir thoroughly, allowing the mixture to cook for 30 seconds before adding the tomato sauce.
5. Pour in the coconut milk and return the shrimp to the skillet, stir well to incorporate.
6. Garnish with fresh cilantro and chili peppers.
7. Serve.

Freestyle Smart Points Per Serving: 2

(Calories 224 | Total Fats 8g | Net Carbs: 9g | Protein 28g | Fiber: 2g)

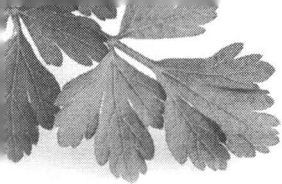

Crispy Shrimp Taquitos

(Prep Time: 15 MIN | Cook Time: 30 MIN | Serves: 6)

Ingredients:

For cooking:

Nonstick spray

1 tsp olive oil

For taquitos:

1 jalapeno (seeded, minced)

2 garlic cloves (peeled, minced)

½ yellow onion (peeled, diced)

1 tomato (diced)

12 ounces fresh shrimp
(peeled, deveined, chopped)

2 tbsp fresh cilantro (finely
chopped)

¼ tsp sea salt

12 low-calorie yellow corn
tortillas

¾ cup pepper jack cheese
(shredded)

Directions:

1. Preheat the main oven to 400 degrees F and cover two baking sheets with aluminum foil. Spritz the foil with nonstick spray.
2. Add the olive oil to a skillet and place over moderate heat.
3. Add the jalapeno, garlic, and onion, sauté for 3-4 minutes until soft.
4. Add the diced tomato and sauté for another few minutes before adding the chopped shrimp, cilantro, and sea salt. Increase the heat to moderately high and sauté for 60 seconds. Take off the heat.
5. Working in batches of four, microwave the tortillas for 30 seconds until soft and warm.
6. Spoon 3 tbsp of filling onto each tortilla and sprinkle with 1 tbsp shredded cheese. Roll up each tortilla like a burrito and arrange on the baking sheets, seam side down.
7. Spritz the taquitos with nonstick spray and place in the oven. Bake for 15 minutes until the tortillas are crispy and golden.

Freestyle Smart Points Per Serving: 5

(Calories 245 | Total Fats 8g | Net Carbs: 24g | Protein 18g | Fiber: 4g)

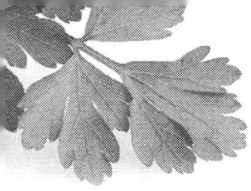

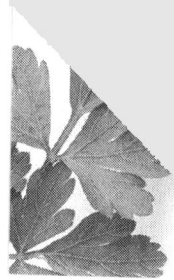

Garlic and Herb Tilapia

(Prep Time: 10 MIN | Cook Time: 8 MIN | Serves: 6)

Ingredients:

For herb and garlic seasoning:

3 tsp olive oil

2 garlic cloves (peeled, crushed)

1 tsp parsley

1 tsp oregano

Kosher salt and black pepper

For fish:

6 (6 ounce) fresh tilapia fillets

2 lemon halves

Directions:

1. Preheat your broiler to a low heat setting.
2. Add all of the seasoning ingredients to a small bowl and stir to combine.
3. Arrange aluminum foil inside a broiler pan and set the tilapia on top. Drizzle the fish evenly with the seasoning and squeeze over the two lemon halves.
4. Arrange the pan several inches away from the flame and cook for 7-8 minutes until cooked through. Serve straight away.

Freestyle Smart Points Per Serving: 1

(Calories 200 | Total Fats 6.5g | Net Carbs: 1.5g | Protein 35g | Fiber: 1g)

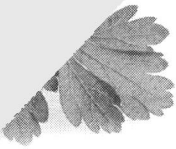

Grilled Lemon and Salmon Kebabs

(Prep Time: 10 MIN | Cook Time: 10 MIN | Serves: 4)

Ingredients:

For cooking:
Nonstick spray

Seasoning:
2 tbsp fresh oregano (finely chopped)

2 tsp sesame seeds

1 tsp cumin

¼ tsp red pepper flakes (crushed)

1 tsp sea salt

For kebabs:
1½ pounds salmon fillet (skin removed, chopped into 1" chunks)

2 lemons (sliced)

8 metal kebab skewers

Directions:

1. Preheat a grill to moderately high heat and spritz the grates with nonstick spray.
2. Add the seasoning to a small bowl and stir to combine. Set to one side.
3. Thread the salmon chunks and lemon slices equally onto the kebab skewers, making sure to begin and end with salmon. Folding the lemon slices in half before skewering.
4. Spritz the kebabs with nonstick spray and sprinkle generously with the seasoning mixture.
5. To cook; grill the fish for 8-9 minutes, turning a few times, on the preheated grill. Enjoy hot.

Freestyle Smart Points Per Serving: 0

(Calories 265 | Total Fats 10g | Net Carbs: 4g | Protein 35g | Fiber: 3g)

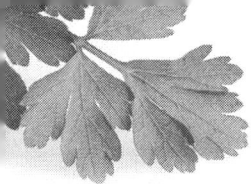

Hot Crab Salad Stuffed Avocado

(Prep Time: 10 MIN | Cook Time: N/A | Serves: 2)

Ingredients:

For crab salad:

2 tsp Asian hot sauce

2 tbsp low-fat mayo

1 tsp fresh chives (chopped)

4 ounces lump crabmeat

¼ cup cucumber (peeled, diced)

For avocado:

1 small, ripe avocado (halved lengthwise, pitted)

½ tsp sesame seeds

2 tsp soy sauce

Directions:

1. Add all of the crab salad ingredients to a small bowl and stir gently but well until combined.
2. Spoon the crab salad into the avocado halves. Sprinkle with sesame seeds and drizzle with soy. Serve straight away.

Freestyle Smart Points Per Serving: 5

(Calories 195 | Total Fats 13g | Net Carbs: 3g | Protein 12g | Fiber: 4g)

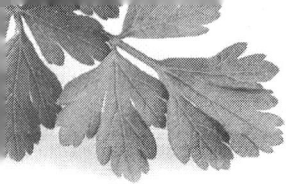

Mussels in White Wine and Basil Cream

(Prep Time: 10 MIN | Cook Time: 20 MIN | Serves: 3)

Ingredients:

For cooking:

2 tsp salted butter

For mussels:

1 garlic clove (peeled, finely chopped)

1 shallot (minced)

½ cup dry white wine

2 pounds fresh mussels (scrubbed, debearded, unopened mussels discarded)

¼ cup fat-free half & half

For sauce:

¼ cup fat-free half & half

2 garlic cloves (peeled, smashed)

2 tbsp olive oil

¼ cup Parmesan cheese (grated)

½ cup fresh basil leaves

Sea salt and black pepper

Directions:

1. First, prepare the mussels. In a deep saucepan, melt the butter. Add the garlic and shallot, sauté for 3-4 minutes. Pour in the wine and heat until boiling.

2. Add the mussels and cook, covered, for approximately 5 minutes until the mussels 'pop' open.

3. Transfer the cooked mussels to a serving bowl leaving the sauce behind in the pan. Discard any mussels that have not properly opened.

4. Add the half & half to the pan and bring to a simmer for 4-5 minutes.

5. In the meantime, add all of the sauce ingredients to a blender and blitz until pureed, add to the pan.

6. Stir the sauce in the pan well, while cooking for another 3-4 minutes. When hot-through, pour over the cooked mussels and serve straight away.

Freestyle Smart Points Per Serving: 7

(Calories 370 | Total Fats 24g | Net Carbs: 11.5g | Protein 20.5g | Fiber: 0.5g)

INSTANT POT
SEAFOOD DISHES

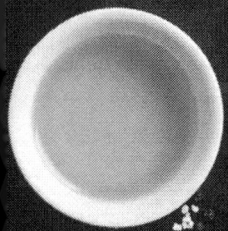

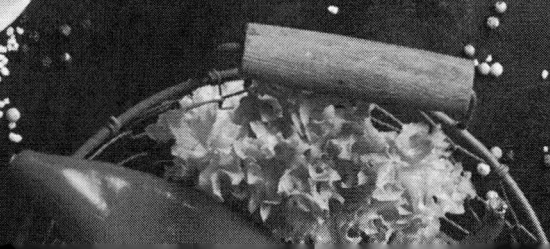

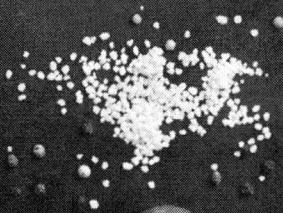

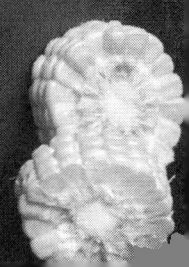

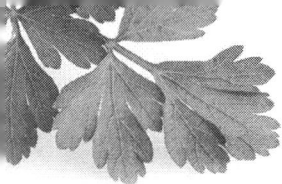

Shrimp Scampi with Cucumber Dill Sauce

(Prep Time: 5 MIN | Cook Time: 7 MIN | Serves: 2)

Ingredients:

For cooking:

Nonstick spray

For shrimp scampi:

4 oz shrimps, cleaned and deveined

½ cup broccoli, chopped

1 small carrot, sliced

1 small onion, finely chopped

1 garlic clove, finely chopped

½ tsp sea salt

¼ tsp cayenne pepper, ground

For cucumber dill sauce:

½ cup cucumber, sliced

1 tsp mayonnaise, fat-free

1 tsp fresh dill, finely chopped

½ tsp garlic powder

¼ tsp dried thyme, ground

½ tsp salt

½ tsp black pepper, ground

Directions:

1. In a food processor or a blender, combine cucumber, mayonnaise, dill, garlic powder, dried thyme, salt, and pepper. Pulse until smooth and creamy. Set aside.

2. Plug in your Instant Pot and press the Sauté button. Spray with some non-stick cooking spray and add onions and garlic. Stir-fry for 3-4 minutes, or until the onions are translucent. Add shrimps and sprinkle with sea salt and cayenne pepper. Cook for 1 minute, turning once.

3. Add broccoli and carrot. Securely lock the lid and adjust the steam release handle. Press the Manual button and cook for 2 minutes on High pressure.

4. When done, perform a quick pressure release and open the pot. Drain the ingredients and transfer to a large colander.

5. Drizzle with cucumber dill sauce and serve immediately. Enjoy!

Freestyle SmartPoints Per Serving: 6

(Calories 242 | Total Fats 4g | Net Carbs: 17.9g | Protein 29.5g | Fiber: 5g)

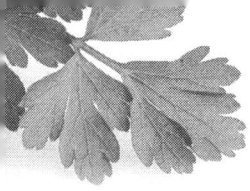

Salmon Risotto

(Prep Time: 5 MIN | Cook Time: 10 MIN | Serves: 3)

Ingredients:

For cooking:
2 tsp olive oil

For risotto:
1 cup cauliflower florets, finely chopped

7 oz salmon fillets

1 large tomato, roughly chopped

1 red bell pepper, sliced

¼ cup green peas

2 medium-sized celery stalk, chopped

Seasoning:
2 tsp Cajun seasoning

½ tsp white pepper, ground

Directions:

1. Plug in the Instant Pot and add olive oil to the stainless steel insert. Heat on Sauté mode and add salmon, tomato, red bell pepper, green peas, and celery. Stir-fry for 3-4 minutes and then add 1 cup of water.

2. Bring it to a boil and add cauliflower. Cook for 5 more minutes, stirring occasionally.

3. Sprinkle with Cajun seasoning and white pepper. Optionally, add some salt and chili pepper for spicier taste.

4. Turn off the pot and transfer to a serving plate.

5. Optionally, sprinkle with some fresh chives or finely chopped spring onions. Enjoy!

Freestyle SmartPoints Per Serving: 4

(Calories 160 | Total Fats 7.5g | Net Carbs: 6.6g | Protein 15.3g | Fiber: 3.1g)

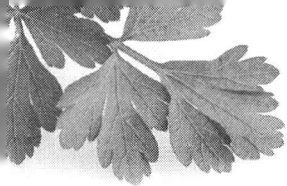

Crab Parsley Patties

(Prep Time: 15 MIN | Cook Time: 13 MIN | Serves: 6)

Ingredients:

For cooking:

Nonstick cooking spray

For patties:

1 lb crab meat

½ cup fresh parsley, finely chopped

1 small red onion, finely chopped

3 large eggs, lightly beaten

2 tsp dry sherry

½ cup panko breadcrumbs

1 tsp butter

Seasoning:

1 tsp salt

¼ tsp black pepper, ground

¼ tsp garlic powder

Directions:

1. Plug in the Instant Pot and press the Sauté button. Add butter and gently stir with a wooden spatula until melts.
2. Add onions and stir-fry for 4-5 minutes, or until lightly caramelized. Remove to a large bowl and turn off the pot.
3. Add crab meat, parsley, eggs, sherry, salt, pepper, and garlic powder to the bowl with onions. Mix well with your hands and form the patties, about 3-inch in diameter. Roll in breadcrumbs and transfer to baking sheet. Refrigerate for 20 minutes.
4. Spray the inner pot with some cooking spray and press the Sauté button. Cook patties 3-4 minutes on each side, or until nicely browned. Enjoy!

Freestyle SmartPoints Per Serving: 5

(Calories 155 | Total Fats 4.1g | Net Carbs: 13.5g | Protein 9.4g | Fiber: 0.8g)

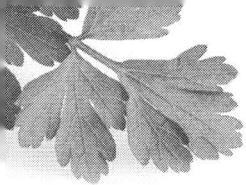

Lemon Tuna with Herbs

(Prep Time: 5 MIN | Cook Time: 7 MIN | Serves: 4)

Ingredients:

For cooking:
2 tsp olive oil

For lemon tuna:
1 lb tuna fillets, cut into bite-
sized pieces

1 whole lemon, thinly sliced

1 medium-sized red bell
pepper, chopped

1 tbsp fresh parsley, finely
chopped

½ tsp sea salt

¼ tsp black pepper, ground

Herbs:
1 fresh rosemary sprig

1 tsp fresh thyme, finely
chopped

1 tsp fresh sage, finely
chopped

Directions:

1. Grease the stainless steel insert of your Instant Pot with some cooking spray. Add chopped tuna and sprinkle with some salt and pepper. Cook for 1 minute on each side and then add bell pepper. Stir-fry for 2-3 minutes.

2. Now, pour 1 cup of water and add all the remaining ingredients and herbs. Stir once and securely lock the lid.

3. Set the steam release handle and press the Manual button. Set the timer for 2 minutes and cook on High pressure.

4. When you hear the cookers end signal, perform a quick pressure release by moving the valve to the Venting position. Open the pot and drain the tuna and pepper.

5. Transfer to a serving plate and garnish with some fresh lemon. Enjoy!

Freestyle SmartPoints Per Serving: 2

(Calories 145 | Total Fats 3.7g | Net Carbs: 1.9g | Protein 25.3g | Fiber: 0.5g)

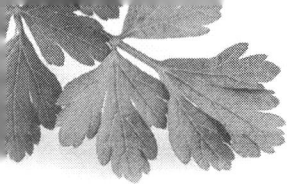

Shrimps in Honey Mirin Sauce

(Prep Time: 5 MIN | Cook Time: 8 MIN | Serves: 4)

Ingredients:

For cooking:
1 cup fish stock

For shrimps:
1 lb shrimps, peeled and deveined
1 tbsp spring onions, finely chopped

For honey wasabi sauce:
1 tbsp honey
2 tbsp mirin
½ tsp wasabi paste
1 tbsp soy sauce, low-sodium
1 tsp balsamic vinaigrette
½ tsp salt
½ tsp black pepper, ground

Directions:

1. Plug in the Instant Pot and pour in the fish stock. Add shrimps and securely lock the lid. Set the steam release handle by moving the valve to the Sealing position. Press the Manual button and set the timer for 1 minute. Cook on High pressure.
2. When you hear the cookers end signal, release the pressure naturally.
3. Meanwhile, combine all sauce ingredients in a small bowl. Mix until combined.
4. Open the pot and remove the shrimps using a slotted spoon. Reserve the liquid.
5. Press the Sauté button and pour in the sauce. Bring it to a boil and simmer for 5 minutes, stirring occasionally.
6. Turn off the pot and return the shrimps to the pot. Stir once and transfer to a serving dish.
7. Sprinkle with spring onions and serve immediately.

Freestyle SmartPoints Per Serving: 4

(Calories 183 | Total Fats 3.1g | Net Carbs: 10.1g | Protein 27.5g | Fiber: 0.2g)

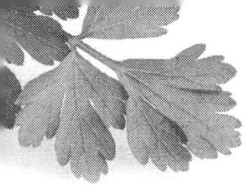

Thai Shrimp Soup

(Prep Time: 10 MIN | Cook Time: 1 HOUR 9 MIN | Serves: 6)

Ingredients:

For cooking:

2 cups chicken broth

For soup:

1 lb whole shrimps

1 cup coconut milk, reduced fat

2-3 lemongrass slices

6 oz oyster mushrooms, sliced

¼ cup fish sauce

2 green chilies, chopped

2 tsp lime juice, fresh

Seasoning:

7 slices fresh ginger

¼ cup parsley leaves, chopped

1 tbsp chili paste

Directions:

1. Plug in the Instant Pot and pour in chicken broth. Press the Sauté button and bring it to a boil. Add lemongrass and ginger. Continue to cook for 2 more minutes.
2. Add oyster mushrooms, coconut milk, and green chilies. Stir well and cook for 2 more minutes.
3. Add shrimps and stir in the fish sauce, lime juice, and chili paste.
4. Securely lock the lid and set the steam release handle by moving the valve to the Sealing position. Set the Slow Cooker mode and cook for 1 hour.
5. When you hear the cookers end signal, release the pressure naturally.
6. Open the pot and transfer the soup to serving bowls. Sprinkle with some fresh parsley and serve warm.

Freestyle SmartPoints Per Serving: 4

(Calories 214 | Total Fats 1.8g | Net Carbs: 15.5g | Protein 27.8g | Fiber: 3.7g)

RED MEAT

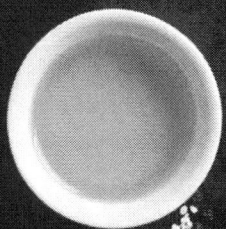
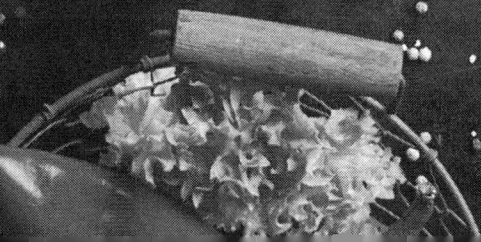
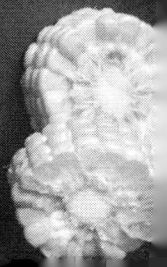

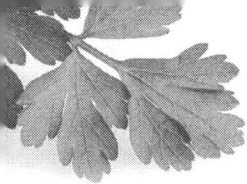

Bacon Wrapped Hot Dogs

(Prep Time: 10 MIN | Cook Time: 20 MIN | Serves: 2)

Ingredients:

For hot dogs:

7 hot dogs (97% fat-free)

7 rashers uncured bacon

Directions:

10. Preheat the main oven to 425 degrees F. Cover a baking sheet with kitchen foil.
11. Wrap a rasher of bacon around each sausage and arrange on the baking sheet.
12. Place in the oven and cook for 15-18 minutes until cooked through and browned.

Freestyle SmartPoints Per Serving: 1

(Calories 75 | Total Fats 3g | Net Carbs: 2g | Protein 11g | Fiber: 0g)

RED MEAT

Beef and Ricotta Meatballs with Sage

(Prep Time: 10 MIN | Cook Time: 20 MIN | Serves: 8)

Ingredients:

For cooking:

Nonstick spray

For meatballs:

½ cup fat-free ricotta cheese

1 pound 96% lean ground beef

1 egg

2 tsp sage

4 cloves garlic (peeled, minced)

Sea salt and black pepper

2 cups Panko breadcrumbs

Directions:

1. Preheat the main oven to 325 degrees F. Cover a baking sheet with parchment and spritz with nonstick spray.
2. Add all of the meatball ingredients (excluding the breadcrumbs) to a large bowl, and, using clean hands, mix until well combined.
3. Add the Panko breadcrumbs to a small bowl.
4. Roll the meat mixture into 24 equally sized balls and roll each ball in the breadcrumbs, before placing on the parchment lined baking sheet.
5. Place in the oven and bake for just over 15 minutes, until sufficiently cooked.

Freestyle SmartPoints Per Serving: 3

(Calories 125 | Total Fats 3g | Net Carbs: 8g | Protein 15g | Fiber: 0g)

Cheesy Garlic Potato Patties with Bacon

(Prep Time: 10 MIN | Cook Time: 25 MIN | Serves: 10)

Ingredients:

For cooking:
Nonstick spray

For patties:
4 tbsp cooked crispy bacon (crumbled)

1½ cups prepared mashed potato (cool)

½ tsp powdered garlic

⅓ cup low-fat Cheddar cheese (grated)

For coating:
½ cup Panko breadcrumbs

1 tbsp Parmesan cheese (grated)

White of 1 medium egg

Directions:

1. Preheat the main oven to 400 degrees F. Spritz a baking sheet with nonstick spray.
2. Add all of the patty ingredients to a large bowl and mix well until combined.
3. Combine the breadcrumbs and Parmesan in a bowl.
4. Taking a ¼ cup of potato mixture at a time, form into patties, brushing each with egg white on both sides and then coating in the breadcrumb mixture and arranging on the baking sheet.
5. Place in the oven and bake for 25 minutes, flipping the patties halfway through cooking.
6. Allow to cool and set a little, before serving warm.

Freestyle SmartPoints Per Serving: 2

(Calories 65 | Total Fats 2g | Net Carbs: 10g | Protein 3g | Fiber: 0.5g)

RED MEAT

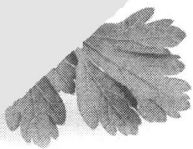

Chinese Beef in Orange Sauce

(Prep Time: 10 MIN | Cook Time: 20 MIN | Serves: 4)

Ingredients:

For cooking:
1 tsp olive oil

For beef:
¾ cup brown rice

1 pound lean sirloin steak
(sliced into strips)

1 yellow onion (peeled,
sliced)

1 tsp olive oil

4 cloves garlic (peeled,
minced)

Sea salt and black pepper

For sauce:
½ tsp grated orange zest

Juice of 1 small orange

¼ cup soy sauce

1 tsp sesame oil

1 tbsp cornstarch

Directions:

1. Cook the rice according to packet directions. Drain and set to one side.
2. Add all of the sauce ingredients to a small bowl and whisk until combined.
3. To a larger bowl, add the strips of steak and all remaining beef ingredients, tossing until combined.
4. Heat the olive oil in a skillet and place over moderately high heat.
5. Add the steak mixture and sauté for 5-6 minutes before pouring in the sauce.
6. Cook, while stirring, for a few minutes, until the sauce becomes thick and is heated through. Serve over rice.

Freestyle SmartPoints Per Serving: 11

(Calories 410 | Total Fats 10g | Net Carbs: 34g | Protein 38g | Fiber: 2g)

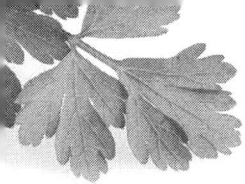

Italian Steak Pizzaiola

(Prep Time: 15 MIN | Cook Time: 20 MIN | Serves: 4)

Ingredients:

For cooking:
Nonstick spray
2 tsp olive oil

For vegetables:
8 ounces fresh mushrooms (sliced)
1 tbsp garlic (peeled, minced)
1 bell pepper (deseed, sliced)
1 cup yellow onion (peeled, finely chopped)

For sauce:
28 ounces canned diced tomatoes
1 tsp granulated sugar
1 tbsp tomato paste
¼ tsp red pepper flakes
2 tsp Italian seasoning
2 tbsp balsamic vinegar

For steak:
1 pound extra lean sirloin steaks
2 tbsp Worcestershire sauce
Salt and black pepper

Directions:

1. Spritz a skillet with nonstick spray and add the oil, place over moderately high heat.
2. Add the vegetables and sauté for 5 minutes, until softened.
3. Add all of the sauce ingredients to the skillet and cook for 5-6 minutes, while stirring, until the sauce thickens. Turn down to low heat and keep warm while you prepare the steak.
4. Spritz a second pan with nonstick spray and place over moderately high heat.
5. Season the steaks with Worcestershire sauce, salt, and pepper, then arrange in the pan and cook for approximately 5 minutes each side.
6. Set the steak aside for 5 minutes to rest and then slice into medium strips.
7. Serve the steak topped with the sauce.

Freestyle SmartPoints Per Serving: 5

(Calories 255 | Total Fats 8g | Net Carbs: 14g | Protein 28g | Fiber: 3g)

RED MEAT

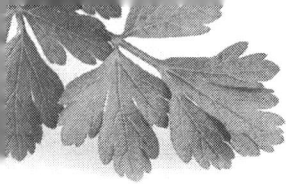

Persian Kabobs

(Prep Time: 15 MIN | Cook Time: 10 MIN | Serves: 4)

Ingredients:

For cooking:
Nonstick spray

For kabobs:
3 cloves garlic (peeled, minced)

1 pound 96% lean ground beef

1 tsp ground sumac

1 yellow onion (peeled, grated)

¼ cup liquid egg substitute

½ cup whole wheat breadcrumbs

1 tsp turmeric

1 tsp sweet paprika

Sea salt and black pepper

Directions:

1. Preheat the main oven to 400 degrees F.
2. Add all of the kabob ingredients to a large bowl and mix thoroughly, using clean hands, until combined.
3. Shape the kabob mixture into 8, 4½" long cigars and arrange on a grill pan.
4. Grill for approximately 4 minutes on each side until cooked through and serve hot.

Freestyle SmartPoints Per Serving: 6

(Calories 240 | Total Fats 7g | Net Carbs: 13g | Protein 29g | Fiber: 1g)

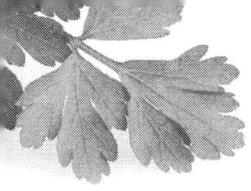

Rosemary and Garlic Rack of Lamb

(Prep Time: 1 HOUR 15 MIN | Cook Time: 25 MIN | Serves: 4)

Ingredients:

For cooking:

Nonstick spray

For rub:

1 tsp fresh thyme (finely chopped)

2 tsp fresh rosemary (finely chopped)

Sea salt and black pepper

2 garlic cloves (peeled, minced)

2 tbsp olive oil

For lamb:

1 (2½ pound) rack Frenched lamb

Directions:

1. Add all rub ingredients to a small bowl and stir to combine.
2. Arrange the rack of lamb on a baking sheet and rub it well with the herb/oil mixture. Allow to sit at room temperate for 60 minutes.
3. Preheat the main oven to 450 degrees F.
4. Place the lamb in the oven and roast for 15 minutes, before rotating the baking sheet 180 degrees and cooking for a further 10 minutes.
5. Allow the lamb to rest for 10 minutes before slicing and serving.

Freestyle SmartPoints Per Serving: 10

(Calories 295 | Total Fats 25g | Net Carbs: 0g | Protein 16g | Fiber: 0g)

RED MEAT

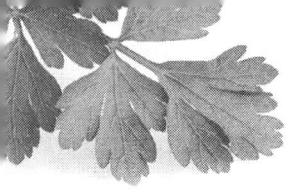

Tamale Pie

(Prep Time: 15 MIN | Cook Time: 50 MIN | Serves: 8)

Ingredients:

For cooking:
Nonstick cooking spray

For cornbread topping:
1½ cups cold water
1 (16 ounce) package low-fat South-western cornbread mix

For tamale filling:
1 pound extra lean ground beef
2 cups onions (peeled, chopped)
1 tbsp fresh garlic (peeled, minced)
1 (15 ounce) can black beans (rinsed, drained)
1 cup fresh corn kernels
1 (14 ½ ounce) can diced tomatoes in juice
1/3 cup reduced-fat Cheddar cheese (grated)
2 tbsp chili powder
½ tsp salt
Freshly ground black pepper

Directions:

1. Preheat the main oven to 375 degrees F. Spritz a 9" baking dish with nonstick spray.
2. First, prepare the tamale filling. In a large frying pan over moderate heat, add the ground beef along with the onions and garlic. Cook, while stirring frequently, using the back of a spoon to break the meat up while it browns. Drain the mixture, using a colander and return to the pan.
3. Add the beans, corn kernels, tomatoes in juice, grated cheese, and chili powder. Stir for 4-5 minutes to combine and season to taste. Remove from the heat.
4. Next, make the cornbread topping: In a mixing bowl, combine the water with the cornbread mix. Gently blend by hand, until lump-free.
5. Transfer the tamale mixture to the baking dish, spreading the mixture evenly.
6. Evenly spread the cornbread batter on top of the tamale mixture.
7. Bake in the oven for 30-35 minutes until springy to the touch.
8. Allow to cool and slice.
9. Enjoy.

Freestyle SmartPoints Per Serving: 10

(Calories 380 | Total Fats 9g | Net Carbs: 52g | Protein 21g | Fiber: 4g)

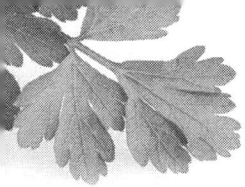

Beef and Spinach Noodle Rolls

(Prep Time: 15 MIN | Cook Time: 40 MIN | Serves: 6)

Ingredients:

For cooking:

2 tsp virgin olive oil

Nonstick spray

For lasagne:

6 wholewheat lasagne noodles

½ pound lean ground beef

½ pound crimini mushrooms (roughly chopped)

2 cloves garlic (peeled, minced)

5 ounces fresh baby spinach

½ cup part-skim ricotta cheese

¼ cup fresh basil (chopped)

3 tbsp Parmesan cheese (chopped)

1 (15-ounce) jar fat-free marinara sauce

Directions:

1. Cook the noodles according to the package instructions, until al dente. Drain and rinse.

2. In a large frying pan heat the olive oil over moderately high heat. Add the ground beef followed by the mushrooms and garlic. Using the back of a wooden spoon break up the meat, while occasionally stirring until the mushrooms are fork-tender, 8-10 minutes.

3. Add the spinach and cook, while constantly stirring, until the spinach wilts, 2-3 minutes.

4. Transfer the mixture to a mixing bowl, and allow to cool a little. Add the ricotta cheese, chopped basil, followed by 2 tbsp of Parmesan cheese, stirring well until combined.

5. Preheat the main oven to 350 degrees F. Spritz a 9" square casserole dish with nonstick spray.

6. Spread ½ cup of marinara sauce over the bottom of the casserole dish.

7. Ensure the cooked noodles are dry and arrange on a clean work surface.

8. Evenly spread the beef mixture over the noodles and beginning with the short end, carefully roll up as you would a jelly roll and place in the casserole dish, seam side facing down.

9. Pour the remaining marinara sauce over the rolls. Cover loosely with aluminum foil and bake in the oven until bubbling, for approximately half an hour.

10. Garnish with the remaining Parmesan cheese and enjoy.

Freestyle Smart Points Per Serving: 7

(Calories 253 | Total Fats 7g | Net Carbs: 22g | Protein 18g | Fiber: 6g)

RED MEAT

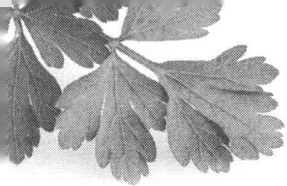

Chinese Braised Beef

(Prep Time: 8 HOUR 15 MIN | Cook Time: 6 HOUR | Serves: 6)

Ingredients:

For marinade:

⅔ cup soy sauce

½ cup sake

2 garlic cloves (peeled, minced)

½ tsp freshly ground black pepper

2 tbsp sugar

For beef:

1¾ pounds chuck roast (fat trimmed, cut into 1" pieces)

2 cups onions (peeled, coarsely chopped)

1 cup chicken broth

2 tbsp cornstarch mixed with ¼ cup chicken broth

½ pound shitake mushrooms (stems removed, caps sliced)

10 ounces baby spinach

Directions:

1. In a large bowl, whisk together all of the marinade ingredients.
2. Add the chuck roast to the marinade and stir to coat evenly. Cover the bowl and chill overnight.
3. Transfer the meat along with the marinade to a 5-6 quart slow cooker along with the onions and chicken broth, on high, cook for between 3-4 hours.
4. Skim off any surface fat and add the cornstarch-chicken broth mixture, stirring to incorporate. Add the mushrooms followed by the baby spinach.
5. Cover and on low, cook for another 1-2 hours until the meat is fork tender and the sauce thickened.
6. Serve.

Freestyle Smart Points Per Serving: 6

(Calories 232 | Total Fats 8g | Net Carbs: 17g | Protein 40g | Fiber: 3g)

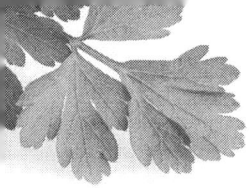

Lamb Stroganoff

(Prep Time: 15 MIN | Cook Time: 8 HOUR | Serves: 8)

Ingredients:

For cooking:

1 tbsp extra virgin olive oil

For cream sauce:

1 cup light sour cream

1/3 cup all-purpose flour

¼ cup dry sherry

For serving:

¼ cup Italian flat-leaf parsley (chopped)

1 (12-ounce) pack dried wholegrain wide noodles (cooked)

For lamb:

1¾ pounds boneless lamb sirloin (fat trimmed, cut into 1" chunks)

34 cup low-sodium beef broth

4 cups white mushrooms (sliced)

2 cups sweet onions (sliced)

1 tbsp Dijon mustard

3 garlic cloves (peeled, minced)

1 bay leaf

½ tsp sea salt

¼ tsp freshly ground black pepper

Directions:

1. In a large skillet over moderately high heat, add the oil and brown the lamb. Drain away any excess fat.
2. Transfer the browned lamb to a crock pot along with all remaining lamb ingredients.
3. Cover with the lid, and on low heat, cook for between 6-8 hours.
4. In a medium-sized mixing bowl, whisk together the cream sauce ingredients until totally combined. Stir approximately ½ a cup of hot liquid from the crockpot into the cream sauce. Transfer the mixture to the crockpot and stir well.
5. Re-cover the crock pot and on a high heat setting cook for half an hour, or until the sauce is bubbling and thick.
6. Remove and discard the bay leaf.
7. Add the chopped parsley, stir to combine and serve with cooked noodles.

Freestyle Smart Points Per Serving: 9

(Calories 373 | Total Fats 10g | Net Carbs: 35g | Protein 31g | Fiber: 5g)

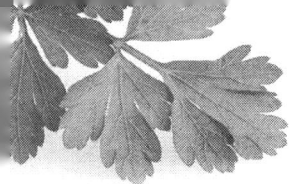

Mexican Beef Enchilada Casserole

(Prep Time: 20 MIN | Cook Time: 40 MIN | Serves: 8)

Ingredients:

For cooking:

Nonstick spray

Garnish:

Fresh tomato (chopped)

Scallions (chopped)

For enchiladas:

1 medium onion (peeled, chopped)

2 garlic cloves (peeled, pressed)

1 pound extra-lean ground beef

2 tbsp low-sodium taco seasoning mix

1 (11 ounce) can Mexican corn (drained)

1 (12 ounce) jar chunky salsa

1 (14 ounce) can non-fat refried beans

3 tbsp water

6 (6") corn tortillas

1 cup low-fat Mexican style cheese

Directions:

1. Preheat the main oven to 400 degrees F.
2. Spritz a large frying pan set over moderate heat with nonstick spray.
3. Add the onion, followed by the garlic and ground beef to the pan, using the back of a wooden spoon to break up the meat. Cook until the meat is gently browned all over and the onion softened. Drain away any excess fat from the mixture.
4. Add the taco seasoning, and corn along with 1 cup of the salsa and mix to combine.
5. In a mixing bowl, combine the refried beans with the water until spreadable and smooth.
6. To assemble, spritz a 9x13" casserole dish with nonstick spray. Arrange 2 tortillas over the base of the casserole dish. Cut one of the tortillas to fill any available gaps as you assemble each layer. Evenly spread a ⅓ of the beans over the tortillas. Top with a ⅓ of the beef mixture and a ⅓ of the cheese. Repeat. Lay the other 2 tortillas on top of the cheese and top with the remaining refried beans and meat mixture.
7. Cover with aluminum foil and bake in the preheated oven until hot, this will take around 25 minutes. Remove the aluminum foil and evenly top with the remaining salsa and cheese. Bake for another 7-10 minutes, or until the cheese is totally melted.
8. Remove from the oven and put to one side for several minutes before serving. Garnish with tomatoes and scallions.
9. Serve.

Freestyle Smart Points Per Serving: 4

(Calories 298 | Total Fats 9g | Net Carbs: 22.5g | Protein 26.8g | Fiber: 5.5g)

Mustard Pork Tenderloin with Apple

(Prep Time: 10 MIN | Cook Time: 8 HOUR | Serves: 6)

Ingredients:

For cooking:
Nonstick spray

For pork:
2 pound lean pork tenderloin
(fat removed)
1½ tsp kosher salt
½ tsp black pepper
2 tbsp wholegrain mustard
2 tbsp runny honey
1 onion (peeled, thinly sliced)
2 apples (cored, sliced)

Directions:

1. Spritz a slow cooker with nonstick spray.
2. Season the pork tenderloin with kosher salt and black pepper and add to the slow cooker.
3. Evenly spread the wholegrain mustard and runny honey on the tenderloin.
4. Cover with slices of onions and apples.
5. Cook in the slow cooker for between 6-8 hours.
6. Remove the lid from the slow cooker for the final half an hour; this will allow the liquid to reduce.
7. Slice the pork and enjoy.

Freestyle Smart Points Per Serving: 3

(Calories 232 | Total Fats 4g | Net Carbs: 15g | Protein 32g | Fiber: 2g)

RED MEAT

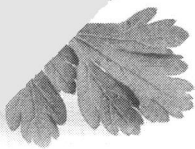

Party Ham with Honey Mustard and Orange

(Prep Time: 10 MIN | Cook Time: 6 HOUR | Serves: 20)

Ingredients:

For cooking:
Nonstick spray

For ham:
1 (6-7 pound) bone-in, spiral cut ham (fully cooked)
1 cup ginger ale

For the rub:
¼ cup runny honey
2 tbsp spicy brown mustard
¼ tsp ground ginger
¼ tsp ground cloves
¼ tsp ground cinnamon
Juice of 1 medium orange

Directions:

1. Place the ham, unwrapped, into a 6-7 quart slow cooker, flat side facing down.
2. In a mixing bowl, combine the rub ingredients, stirring to incorporate. Rub the mixture all over the cooked ham.
3. Pour the ginger ale over the top of the ham.
4. Cover the slow cooker, and on low, cook for between 4-6 hours, until the ham is sufficiently heated.
5. Remove the ham from the slow cooker and place on a chopping board. Allow to rest for several minutes before slicing.

Freestyle Smart Points Per Serving: 6

(Calories 140 | Total Fats 7g | Net Carbs: 2g | Protein 16g | Fiber: 0g)

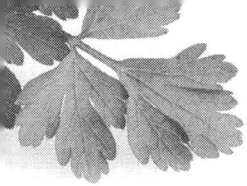

Pork Chops with Mustard Sauce

(Prep Time: 15 MIN | Cook Time: 20 MIN | Serves: 4)

Ingredients:

For cooking:
1 tsp butter

For chops:
4 (5½ ounce) pork chops
(trimmed of fat, 1"thick)
3 tbsp onion (peeled, chopped)
¾ cup chicken stock
1 tbsp Dijon mustard
2 tbsp parsley (chopped)
Dash pepper

Seasoning:
½ tsp sea salt
Freshly ground black pepper

Directions:

1. In a large frying pan melt the butter over a moderately low heat.
2. Season the pork chops.
3. Increase the heat to moderate and add the pork chops to the frying pan and sauté for 6-8 minutes. Flip and cook until the pork chops are browned and medium, approximately 6-8 minutes longer. Set the cooked pork to one side.
4. Add the onion to the frying pan and cook, while stirring for 2-3 minutes, until softened. Pour in the stock and boil until it reduces to approximately ½ a cup, for 2-3 minutes.
5. Stir in the Dijon mustard, parsley, and a dash of pepper.
6. Arrange the cooked chops on a serving platter. Pour the mustard sauce over the meat.

Freestyle Smart Points Per Serving: 5

(Calories 180 | Total Fats 5g | Net Carbs: 1g | Protein 29g | Fiber: 0g)

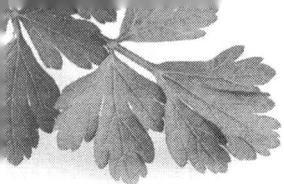

Sirloin Steak with Homemade Chimichurri

(Prep Time: 10 MIN | Cook Time: 10 MIN | Serves: 4)

Ingredients:

For chimichurri:

2 tbsp olive oil

1 tbsp red vinegar

1 tbsp water

2 tbsp fresh parsley

2 tbsp fresh cilantro

2 tbsp fresh basil

1 garlic clove (peeled, minced)

Salt and pepper

For steak:

1⅓ pounds lean sirloin steak (trimmed of fat)

1 tsp sea salt

½ tsp freshly ground black pepper

½ tsp cumin

½ tsp garlic powder

Directions:

1. Preheat a grill to moderate heat for direct cooking.
2. Prepare the chimichurri; add all of the chimichurri ingredients to a food processor and blitz until smooth and combined. Add a drop more water if necessary.
3. Rub the steak all over with the sea salt, black pepper, cumin and garlic powder.
4. Grill the steak to your preferred level of doneness (approximately 4-5 minutes each side for medium rare). Remove the steak from the grill and allow to rest.
5. Slice the steak against the grain and serve with chimichurri.

Freestyle Smart Points Per Serving: 5

(Calories 280 | Total Fats 19g | Net Carbs: 1g | Protein 25g | Fiber: 0g)

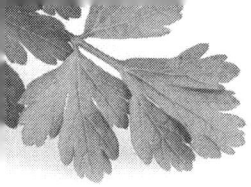

Philly Cheesesteak Mushrooms

(Prep Time: 15 MIN | Cook Time: 30 MIN | Serves: 4)

Ingredients:

For cooking:
Nonstick spray

For steak mushrooms:
4 Portobello mushrooms

Sea salt and black pepper

6 ounces sirloin steak (sliced into thin strips)

¾ cup green bell pepper (seeded, diced)

¾ cup yellow onion (peeled, diced)

For cheese sauce:
¼ cup low-fat sour cream

2 tbsp low-fat mayo

2 ounces low-fat cream cheese (at room temperature)

3 ounces low-fat Cheddar cheese (shredded)

Directions:

1. Preheat the main oven to 400 degrees F. Spritz a baking tray with nonstick spray.
2. First, prepare the mushrooms. Remove their stems and gills then spritz with nonstick spray and season with sea salt and black pepper. Set to one side.
3. Season the steak strips with sea salt and black pepper.
4. Spritz a skillet with nonstick spray and place over high heat. Add the steak to the skillet and sauté for 60-90 seconds on each side until cooked. Transfer to a plate.
5. Spritz the same skillet with more nonstick spray and place over moderately low heat.
6. Add the bell pepper and onion to the skillet and sauté for 5 minutes until soft. Take off the heat and set to one side.
7. Add all of the cheese sauce ingredients to a medium bowl and stir until well combined. Add the strips of steak, cooked peppers, and onion to the cheese mixture.
8. Arrange the mushroom caps on the baking tray and stuff each with half a cup of the cheesesteak mixture.
9. Place in the oven and bake for 20 minutes until the cheesesteak mixture is melted and bubbling.
10. Serve hot.

Freestyle Smart Points Per Serving: 7

(Calories 255 | Total Fats 16g | Net Carbs: 6g | Protein 20g | Fiber: 4g)

INSTANT POT
RED MEAT DISHES

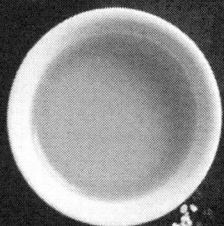

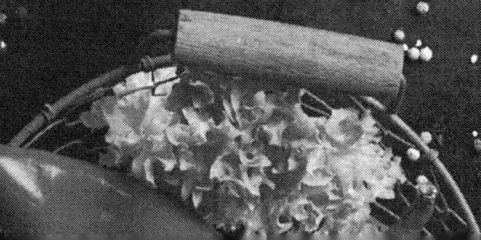

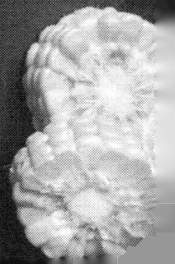

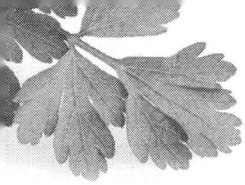

Greek Moussaka

(Prep Time: 15 MIN | Cook Time: 25 MIN | Serves: 6)

Ingredients:

For cooking:
1 tbsp olive oil

For moussaka:
3 eggplants, sliced
1 lb lean ground beef
1 onion, finely chopped
1 garlic clove, crushed
1 cup tomatoes, diced
1 tbsp tomato puree
2 tbsp Parmesan cheese

Seasoning:
1 tsp salt
½ tsp black pepper
1 tsp dried rosemary

Directions:

1. Slice eggplants lengthwise and sprinkle with some salt. Set aside.
2. Plug in the Instant Pot and press the Sauté button. Grease the inner pot with olive oil and heat up. Add onions and garlic and stir-fry for 3-4 minutes.
3. Now add the meat, diced tomatoes, tomato puree, rosemary, and some salt and pepper to taste. Cook for 6-7 minutes, stirring constantly.
4. Press the Cancel button and remove the meat from the pot. Set aside.
5. Rinse the eggplant slices and gently press with your hands. Spread half of the eggplants over a small fitting casserole dish and add the meat. Top with the remaining eggplant slices and sprinkle with parmesan cheese. Optionally, season with some more salt and pepper to taste. Loosely cover with aluminum foil and set aside.
6. Now, set the trivet at the bottom of the inner pot and pour in one cup of water. Place the casserole dish on top and seal the lid.
7. Set the steam release handle to the Sealing position and press the Manual button.
8. Set the timer for 13 minutes on High pressure.
9. When done, perform a quick pressure release and open the lid. Remove the dish from the pot and cool for a while.
10. Slice and serve.

Freestyle SmartPoints Per Serving: 7

(Calories 251 | Total Fats 8.1g | Net Carbs: 9g | Protein 26.9g | Fiber: 10.5g)

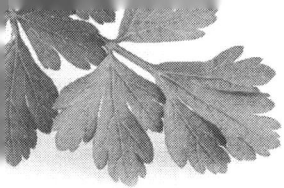

Sriracha Beef Ribs

(Prep Time: 15 MIN | Cook Time: 35 MIN | Serves: 8)

Ingredients:

For cooking:

1 tbsp oil

For beef:

2 lbs beef ribs

2 onions, chopped

3 garlic cloves, crushed

1 cup tomato sauce, sugar-free

4 tbsp sriracha sauce

3 tbsp fish sauce

2 tbsp lime juice

Seasoning:

½ tsp cumin powder

Salt and pepper to taste

Directions:

1. Place ribs in the pot and pour in about 3 cups of water. Sprinkle with some salt and seal the lid.
2. Set the steam release handle to the Sealing position and press the Manual button. Set the timer for 25 minutes on High pressure.
3. When done, perform a quick pressure release and open the lid. Remove the ribs from the pot and chill for a while.
4. Now press the Sauté button and heat the oil.
5. Add onions and garlic. Give it a good stir and cook for 3-4 minutes.
6. Now add the tomato sauce, sriracha, fish sauce, lime juice, and cumin powder. Season with some more salt and pepper to taste and cook for 2 minutes.
7. Add the meat and coat well with the sauce.
8. Press the Cancel button and serve.

Freestyle SmartPoints Per Serving: 5

(Calories 251 | Total Fats 8.9g | Net Carbs: 4.3g | Protein 35.5g | Fiber: 1.1g)

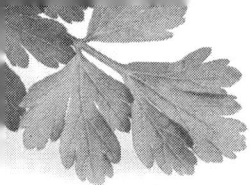

Veal Steaks with Eggplants and Mushrooms

(Prep Time: 10 MIN | Cook Time: 10 MIN | Serves: 4)

Ingredients:

For cooking:

1 tbsp oil

For the steaks:

1lb boneless veal steaks, fat removed

1 cucumber, chopped

½ eggplant, sliced

1 cup button mushrooms

½ purple onion, sliced

2 tbsp soy sauce

1 tbsp mirin

Seasoning:

½ tsp salt

¼ tsp black pepper

¼ tsp dried thyme

Directions:

1. Rinse the meat under cold running water and place on a cutting board. Trim any excess fat and chop into bite-sized pieces. Transfer to a bowl and season with salt, pepper, and thyme. Sprinkle with soy sauce and mix well. Set aside.

2. Plug in the Instant Pot and press the Sauté button. Grease the inner pot with oil and add onions. Cook for 2-3 minutes and then add eggplants. Continue to cook for another 2-3 minutes.

3. Finally, add the meat and mushrooms. Sprinkle with mirin and cook for 5-6 minutes.

4. Press the Cancel button and remove from the pot. Mix with cucumber and serve.

Freestyle SmartPoints Per Serving: 6

(Calories 257 | Total Fats 10.9g | Net Carbs: 7.4g | Protein 29.6g | Fiber: 2.9g)

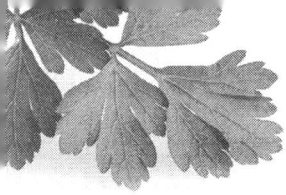

Pulled Pork Nachos

(Prep Time: 20 MIN | Cook Time: 40 MIN | Serves: 8)

Ingredients:

For cooking:
1 tbsp olive oil

Seasoning:
½ tsp salt
¼ tsp black pepper, freshly ground

For pulled pork:
1lb pork shoulder, fat removed
2 large onions, chopped
1 tbsp smoked paprika
1 tsp cayenne pepper
1 tsp garlic powder
½ tsp sugar

For nachos:
½ cup onions, sliced
4 tbsp Cheddar, grated
¼ cup canned corn
4 tbsp BBQ sauce
2 large tortillas, chopped
4 black olives
¼ cup parsley leaves
1 jalapeno pepper, diced

Directions:

1. For the pulled pork, rinse the meat under cold running water and drain in a large colander. Set aside.
2. In a small bowl, mix smoked paprika, cayenne pepper, garlic powder, and sugar. Rub the meat with this mixture and place in the pot. Pour in enough water to cover and add onions. Seal the lid and set the steam release handle to the "Sealing" position. Press the "Manual" button and cook for 30 minutes on High pressure.
3. When done, release the pressure naturally and open the lid. Remove the pork from the pot and place on a cutting board. Cool for a while and shred with two forks. Set aside.
4. Now press the Sauté button and heat up the oil. Add pulled pork and brown for 3-4 minutes. Remove from the pot and set aside.
5. Chop tortillas and place in a small baking dish. Top with onions, corn, pulled pork, diced jalapeno pepper, and olives. Finally, sprinkle with cheese and add some more salt and pepper to taste. Tightly wrap with aluminum foil.
6. Set the trivet at the bottom of the Instant Pot and pour in one cup of water. Add the wrapped pan and seal the lid.
7. Set the steam release handle to the Sealing position and press the Manual button. Set the timer for 5 minutes.
8. When done, perform a quick pressure release and open the lid. Remove the pan and chill for a while.
9. Serve immediately.

Freestyle SmartPoints Per Serving: 4

(Calories 165 | Total Fats 5.8g | Net Carbs: 9.5g | Protein 16.6g | Fiber: 2g)

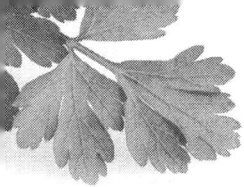

Filet Mignon with Parsley

(Prep Time: 15 MIN | Cook Time: 20 MIN | Serves: 8)

Ingredients:

For filet mignon:

2 filet mignon steaks, about
8oz each

2 tbsp lime juice

2 tbsp Dijon mustard

2 tbsp celery leaves

1 tbsp oil

Seasoning:

1 tsp fresh thyme, finely
chopped

1 tsp onion powder

½ tsp black pepper, freshly
ground

Directions:

1. In a small bowl, combine lime juice, Dijon mustard, oil, celery, thyme, onion powder, and black pepper. Brush fillets with this mixture and refrigerate for 1 hour.

2. Plug in the Instant Pot and set the steam basket. Pour in 1 cup of water.

3. Remove the filets from the refrigerator and place in the basket. Seal the lid and set the steam release handle to the Sealing position.

4. Press the Manual button and set the timer for 15 minutes on high pressure.

5. When done, perform a quick pressure release and open the lid. Remove the filets from the pot and press the Sauté button.

6. Heat up the inner pot and briefly brown filets for 2-3 minutes on each side.

7. Serve immediately.

Freestyle SmartPoints Per Serving: 6

(Calories 178 | Total Fats 13.3g | Net Carbs: 0.1g | Protein 13.6g | Fiber: 0.2g)

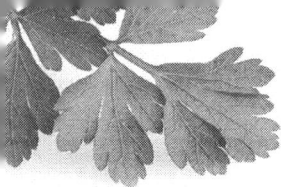

Chili Pork with Roma Tomatoes

(Prep Time: 15 MIN | Cook Time: 35 MIN | Serves: 8)

Ingredients:

For cooking:

1 tbsp oil

2 cups beef stock, low-sodium

For filet mignon:

1 lb pork neck, fat removed and chopped

2 cups Roma tomatoes, whole

2 yellow bell peppers, sliced

1 red bell pepper, sliced

2 green chili peppers, diced

1 cup tomato sauce, sugar-free

¼ cup sweet chili sauce

Seasoning:

Salt and pepper to taste

Directions:

1. Plug in the Instant Pot and grease the inner pot with oil. Press the Sauté button and heat up.
2. Add bell peppers and chili peppers. Cook for 3-4 minutes, stirring constantly. Add Roma tomatoes and cook for another 5 minutes.
3. Now press the Cancel button and stir tomato sauce. Season with some salt and pepper to taste and pour in the stock.
4. Seal the lid and set the steam release handle to the Scaling position. Press the Manual button and cook for 25 minutes on high pressure.
5. When done, perform a quick pressure release and open the lid.
6. Serve immediately.

Freestyle SmartPoints Per Serving: 5

(Calories 213 | Total Fats 6.4g | Net Carbs: 10g | Protein 26.1g | Fiber: 2.4g)

PASTAS & GRAINS

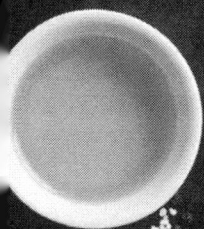

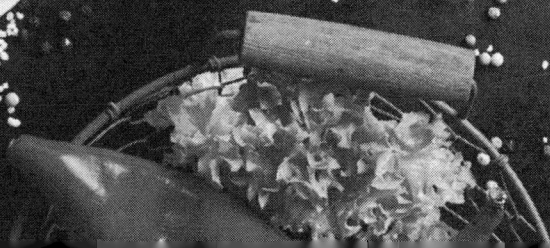

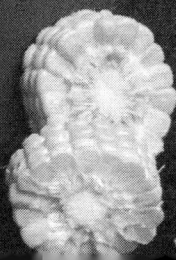

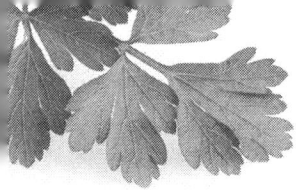

Cajun Jambalaya

(Prep Time: 15 MIN | Cook Time: 1 HOUR | Serves: 6)

Ingredients:

For cooking:

Nonstick spray

1 tsp canola oil

For vegetables:

4 garlic cloves (peeled, minced)

1 yellow onion (peeled, finely chopped)

1 green bell pepper (deseeded, diced)

For jambalaya:

14 ounces smoked turkey sausage (sliced)

1½ pounds skinless, boneless chicken breast (chopped)

1 tbsp Cajun seasoning

1 (14 ounce) can fire-roasted tomatoes

1 tsp celery salt

1 (10½ ounce) can cream of chicken soup (98% fat-free)

1 cup long grain rice

1 cup water

Directions:

1. Preheat the main oven to 375 degrees F and spritz a 13x9" casserole dish with nonstick spray, set to one side.
2. Fry the vegetables in the canola oil in a skillet over moderate heat, until softened.
3. Transfer the cooked vegetables to the casserole dish, along with all of the jambalaya ingredients, stirring well until combined.
4. Cover the dish completely with kitchen foil and place in the oven. Cook for an hour until the chicken is cooked through and the rice is al dente.

Freestyle SmartPoints Per Serving: 6

(Calories 335 | Total Fats 8.5g | Net Carbs: 35.5g | Protein 27g | Fiber: 2.5g)

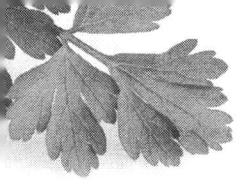

Goat Cheese, Basil, and Lemon Pasta Shells

(Prep Time: 10 MIN | Cook Time: 25 MIN | Serves: 8)

Ingredients:

For cooking:

Nonstick spray

For bake:

1 pound pasta shells

4 cloves garlic (peeled, chopped)

1 pound asparagus (trimmed, chopped)

Sea salt and black pepper

1 tbsp olive oil

1 tbsp freshly grated lemon zest

5 ounces goat's cheese (chopped)

2 tbsp freshly squeezed lemon juice

½ cup fresh basil (chopped)

Directions:

1. Preheat the main oven to 350 degrees F. Cover a baking sheet with kitchen foil and spritz with nonstick spray, then set to one side.

2. Cook the pasta according to packet instructions.

3. In the meantime, arrange the garlic and asparagus on the baking sheet and season with sea salt and black pepper. Place in the oven and cook for just over 10 minutes, until tender.

4. Drain the water from the pasta, reserving 1 cup.

5. Transfer the cooked pasta to a large bowl and drizzle with the olive oil. Scatter over the lemon zest and goat's cheese, followed by the reserved cup of pasta water and lemon juice. Toss to combine.

6. Add the roasted garlic and asparagus, as well as the chopped basil. Season to taste and toss again before serving.

Freestyle SmartPoints Per Serving: 7

(Calories 210 | Total Fats 6g | Net Carbs: 38g | Protein 12g | Fiber: 6g)

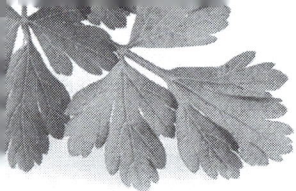

Mexican Corn Casserole

(Prep Time: 15 MIN | Cook Time: 45 MIN | Serves: 6)

Ingredients:

For cooking:

Nonstick spray

For casserole:

1 cup brown rice

1 jalapeno (deseeded, minced)

2 yellow squash (peeled, seeded, diced)

2 cup chicken stock

1½ cups low-fat Mexican cheese (grated)

⅓ cup fresh cilantro (finely chopped)

4 ounces canned green chilies

8 ounces corn

1 cup fat-free sour cream

Sea salt and black pepper

Directions:

1. Preheat the main oven to 350 degrees F and spritz a medium-sized baking dish with nonstick spray and set to one side.
2. Cook the rice according to packet directions and drain.
3. Transfer the cooked rice to the baking dish along with all of the other casserole ingredients. Stir well to combine and place in the oven. Cook for half an hour, until the cheese has melted. Enjoy!

Freestyle SmartPoints Per Serving: 7

(Calories 255 | Total Fats 6g | Net Carbs: 35g | Protein 15g | Fiber: 3g)

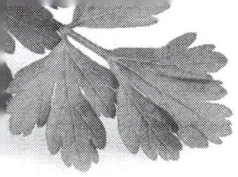

Slow Cooked Chicken Italienne

(Prep Time: 10 MIN | Cook Time: 8 HOURS 10 MIN | Serves: 8)

Ingredients:

For chicken:

8 (5 ounce) skinless, boneless
frozen chicken breasts
2 tsp Italian seasoning
1 (26 ounce) jar tomato-
based pasta sauce
Cooked spaghetti (to serve)

Directions:

1. Add the frozen chicken to your slow cooker.
2. Sprinkle with the Italian seasoning.
3. Pour the tomato-based pasta sauce over the chicken.
4. Cover and cook for 6-8 hours on Low, until the chicken is sufficiently cooked through and its juices run clear.
5. Using 2 metal forks, shred the cooked chicken before serving over spaghetti.

Freestyle SmartPoints Per Serving: 2

(Calories 158 | Total Fats 1.6g | Net Carbs: 4.3g | Protein 28g | Fiber: 2g)

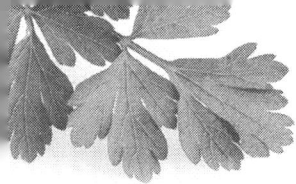

Chili Mac n Cheese

(Prep Time: 10 MIN | Cook Time: 25 MIN | Serves: 8)

Ingredients:

For cooking:

2 tsp olive oil

Seasoning:

2 tsp chili powder

1 tsp cumin

1 tsp sweet paprika

Sea salt and black pepper

For mac n cheese:

1 green bell pepper (diced)

1 red bell pepper (diced)

1 yellow onion (peeled diced)

2 garlic cloves (peeled, minced)

1 pound ground turkey (99% lean)

6 cups reduced-salt chicken stock

1 (20 ounce) can chopped tomatoes with green chilies

1 (14 ounce) can black beans (drained, rinsed)

16 ounces macaroni pasta

¾ cup low-fat Cheddar cheese (shredded)

Directions:

1. Heat the oil in a large saucepan over moderately high heat. Add the red and green peppers and onion and fry for 5 minutes.
2. Add the minced garlic and ground turkey, sauté for 2 minutes before adding the seasoning and stirring well. When the turkey is cooked through, add the chicken stock, chopped tomatoes, and black beans.
3. Bring the mixture to the boil and then toss in the macaroni pasta. Cook for 10-12 minutes until the pasta is soft.
4. Sprinkle with the cheese and allow to stand for 2-3 minutes so that the cheese can melt.
5. Spoon into bowls and serve hot.

Freestyle Smart Points Per Serving: 7

(Calories 360 | Total Fats 10g | Net Carbs: 48g | Protein 30g | Fiber: 10g)

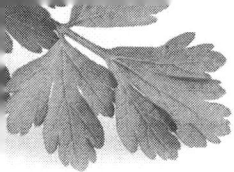

Creamy Cajun Pasta

(Prep Time: 10 MIN | Cook Time: 25 MIN | Serves: 4)

Ingredients:

For cooking:

2 tsp olive oil

For pasta:

8 ounces wholewheat pasta shells

¾ pound skinless, boneless chicken breast (chopped)

1 tbsp Cajun seasoning

1 red bell pepper (sliced into strips)

1 green bell pepper (sliced into strips)

½ red onion (peeled sliced)

4 garlic cloves (peeled, minced)

¼ cup scallions (sliced)

For sauce:

1 (14 ounce) can fire-roasted chopped tomatoes

¼ cup low-fat cream cheese

1 tbsp Cajun seasoning

Sea salt and black pepper

Directions:

1. Cook the pasta according to packet directions. Drain well and set to one side in a large bowl.
2. Add the chopped chicken to a large bowl and toss with 1 tbsp of Cajun seasoning.
3. Heat the olive oil in a skillet and place over moderately high heat, add the chicken to the skillet and sauté for several minutes until cooked. Remove from the skillet and set to one side.
4. To the same skillet, add the pepper strips, onion, and garlic and sauté for several minutes. If they begin to stick, add a splash of water to the skillet.
5. Turn the heat to low and add all of the sauce ingredients to the skillet. Stir well and cook until the cream cheese has melted.
6. Return the cooked chicken and pasta to the skillet and stir well to coat in the sauce.
7. Scatter with scallions and serve hot.

Freestyle Smart Points Per Serving: 8

(Calories 385 | Total Fats 6g | Net Carbs: 45g | Protein 27g | Fiber: 8g)

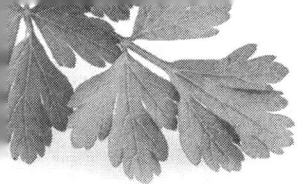

Mushroom and Spinach Lasagna

(Prep Time: 10 MIN | Cook Time: 40 MIN | Serves: 6)

Ingredients:

For cooking:
2 tsp olive oil

For vegetables:
8 cups fresh spinach

4 cloves garlic (peeled, minced)

2 cups fresh mushrooms (peeled, sliced)

1 medium zucchini (chopped)

For white sauce:
1½ cups semi-skim ricotta cheese

1 medium egg

¼ cup Parmesan cheese (shredded)

1½ tsp Italian seasoning mix

Salt and pepper

For lasagna:
1 (28 ounce) jar tomato sauce

12 no-boil lasagne noodle sheets

1 cup semi skim mozzarella cheese (shredded)

Directions:

1. Heat the oil in a skillet and place over moderate heat. Add the vegetables and sauté for 5 minutes, drain away any excess water from the skillet. Cover and cook for 25 minutes.

2. In the meantime, beat together the white sauce ingredients in a medium bowl until combined and set to one side.

3. When the vegetables are cooked, assemble the lasagna; in a clean skillet pour a little of the jarred tomato sauce (just enough to cover the base of the skillet). On top of the sauce, arrange 4 lasagna noodles and then top with a third of the cooked vegetables. Top the vegetables with a third of the white sauce mixture, gently spread the white sauce into an even layer. Repeat this layering twice more.

4. Scatter the shredded mozzarella over the lasagna and place over moderately low heat and cook for just over 20 minutes until the cheese is bubbling.

5. Allow to cool for a few minutes before serving.

Freestyle Smart Points Per Serving: 10

(Calories 347 | Total Fats 13g | Net Carbs: 35g | Protein 21g | Fiber: 5g)

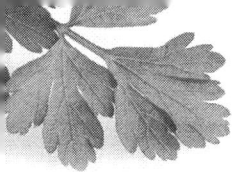

Spanish Paella

(Prep Time: 22 MIN | Cook Time: 40 MIN | Serves: 8)

Ingredients:

For cooking:
2 tsp olive oil

Seasoning:
2 tsp chili powder
1 tsp cumin
1¼ tsp sweet paprika
Sea salt and black pepper

For paella:
½ tsp ground saffron
¼ cup hot water
1 pound uncooked large shrimp (peeled, deveined)
12 ounces chicken chorizo (sliced)
4 medium scallions, white parts (sliced)

1 yellow onion (peeled, finely chopped)
8 ounces cremini mushrooms (sliced)
1 tsp sea salt
1 tbsp garlic (minced)
1 (15-ounce) can chopped tomatoes (drained)

2 cups uncooked Arborio rice
2½ cup canned low-sodium chicken broth
1 cup roasted piquillo peppers (sliced)
1 cup frozen baby peas
¼ cup fresh parsley (chopped)

Directions:

1. In a mixing bowl, combine the ground saffron with the water, stirring to dissolve.
2. In a large skillet over moderately high heat, heat 1 tsp of olive oil. Add the shrimp and cook for 2-3 minutes, each side until opaque. Transfer to a plate.
3. Add the remaining oil followed by the chorizo, scallions, onion, mushrooms, and sea salt; cook while frequently stirring, for 4-6 minutes, until the mushrooms begin to brown.
4. Add the garlic to the skillet, stir a couple of times, and cook for 60 seconds. Add the tomatoes along with the seasoning and Arborio rice, stirring to combine. Pour in the broth and saffron water and heat to boil. Turn the heat down to moderately-low and simmer for 15 minutes.
5. Add the peppers, baby peas, along with the reserved shrimp and continue cooking, uncovered for 5-7 minutes, until the rice is bite tender and is beginning to dry on the bottom of the skillet.
6. Garnish with chopped parsley
7. Serve.

Freestyle Smart Points Per Serving: 8

(Calories 365 | Total Fats 6.5g | Net Carbs: 44g | Protein 27g | Fiber: 4g)

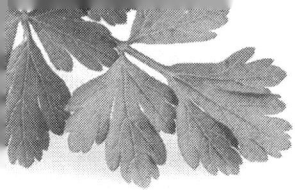

Spicy Sausage and Garlic Penne

(Prep Time: 10 MIN | Cook Time: 20 MIN | Serves: 4)

Ingredients:

For cooking:

1 tbsp olive oil

For penne:

½ yellow onion (peeled, minced)

3 garlic cloves (peeled, minced)

½ pound ground lean turkey sausage

4 cups cauliflower (chopped into small florets)

1 (14 ounce) can chopped tomatoes

8 ounces penne

Seasoning:

1 tsp Italian seasoning mix

1 tsp red pepper flakes

Salt and pepper

Directions:

1. Heat the oil in a skillet and place over moderate heat. Add the minced onion and sauté for 4-5 minutes. Add the garlic and sauté for another 30 seconds.

2. Add the turkey sausage to the skillet and cook for 5 minutes, use a wooden spoon to break up the sausage as it cooks. Add the chopped cauliflower and cook for 5 more minutes, using the wooden spoon to press down on the mixture until it browns.

3. Pour in the chopped tomatoes and seasoning. Stir well and bring to a simmer for 15-18 minutes.

4. While the sauce cooks, prepare the pasta according to packet instructions.

5. Add the cooked pasta to the sauce, stir to combine and serve hot.

Freestyle Smart Points Per Serving: 8

(Calories 342 | Total Fats 15g | Net Carbs: 43g | Protein 20g | Fiber: 9g)

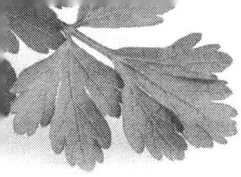

Veggie Alfredo

(Prep Time: 10 MIN | Cook Time: 20 MIN | Serves: 4)

Ingredients:

For cooking:
Nonstick spray

For pasta:
8 ounces pasta

2 tbsp margarine

2 tbsp wholewheat flour

1¼ cups skim milk

½ cup Parmesan cheese (grated)

For vegetables:
1 pound asparagus (trimmed, chopped small)

¼ cup sundried tomatoes (packed in brine/water)

8 ounces fresh mushrooms (peeled, sliced)

2 cups cauliflower (chopped into florets)

4 cloves garlic (peeled, minced)

Seasoning:
Zest of 1 medium lemon

Sea salt and black pepper

Directions:

1. Cook the pasta according to packet directions. Drain well and set to one side in a large bowl.
2. Spritz a skillet with nonstick spray and place over moderately high heat.
3. Add the vegetables to the skillet and sauté for several minutes.
4. In the meantime, melt the margarine in a small saucepan. Sprinkle in the flour and whisk for 60 seconds until lump-free.
5. Pour in the milk and whisk well, cook until the mixture is bubbly and thick.
6. Sprinkle the cheese into the sauce and stir well until it melts and season.
7. Add the cooked vegetables to the cooked pasta and toss well to combine.
8. Pour the hot sauce over the veggie pasta and stir until coated well in the sauce. Spoon into bowls and serve hot.

Freestyle Smart Points Per Serving: 10

(Calories 366 | Total Fats 14g | Net Carbs: 50g | Protein 20g | Fiber: 11g)

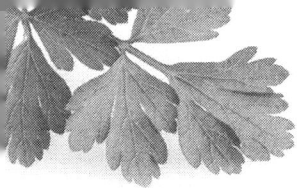

Zesty Lemon Shrimp Spaghetti with Broccoli

(Prep Time: 10 MIN | Cook Time: 20 MIN | Serves: 4)

Ingredients:

For cooking:
2 tsp olive oil

For spaghetti:
8 ounces wholewheat spaghetti

1 pound fresh shrimp (peeled, veined)

1½ cups chicken stock

Juice of 1 medium lemon

4 cloves garlic (peeled, minced)

3 cups broccoli (chopped into florets)

1 (14 ounce) can fire-roasted chopped tomatoes

Salt and pepper

¼ cup Parmesan cheese (grated)

Directions:

1. Cook the spaghetti according to packet instructions, drain and set to one side.
2. Add the oil to a skillet and place over moderately high heat.
3. Sauté the shrimp, for 2 minutes on each side (this may need to be done in batches). Set the shrimp to one side.
4. Add the chicken stock, lemon juice, minced garlic, and broccoli to the skillet. Cook for several minutes until the broccoli is tender.
5. Turn the heat down a little and return the shrimp to the skillet along with the chopped tomatoes and cooked pasta, season well with salt and pepper, and stir. Cook for 2-3 minutes, until hot through.
6. Spoon into bowls and scatter with grated Parmesan.

Freestyle Smart Points Per Serving: 7

(Calories 385 | Total Fats 11g | Net Carbs: 44g | Protein 36g | Fiber: 10g)

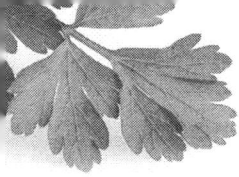

Cheddar Beef Taco Pasta

(Prep Time: 15 MIN | Cook Time: 20 MIN | Serves: 6)

Ingredients:

For pasta:

8 ounces wheat pasta

1 pound 95% lean ground beef

1 (1 ounce) sachet reduced--salt taco seasoning mix

1½ cups chunky salsa

½ cup cold water

¼ cup fat-free sour cream

¾ cup low-fat Cheddar cheese (shredded)

¾ cup sharp Cheddar cheese (shredded)

Salt and pepper (to taste)

Directions:

1. Cook the pasta according to the package directions

2. In the meantime, and while the pasta cooks, add the ground beef to a frying pan and over moderately high heat, using a wooden spoon break the meat up, cook until browned all over.

3. Drain the grease from the pan and add the taco seasoning mix, chunky salsa, and water. Reduce the heat, and simmer until the pasta has finished cooking, for approximately 4-5 minutes.

4. As soon as the pasta is cooked, drain and add it to the beef. Pour in the sour cream, and add the cheese. Season with salt and pepper and stir to incorporate.

5. When the cheese has melted, remove from the heat and serve.

Freestyle Smart Points Per Serving: 10

(Calories 376 | Total Fats 13g | Net Carbs: 31g | Protein 29g | Fiber: 6g)

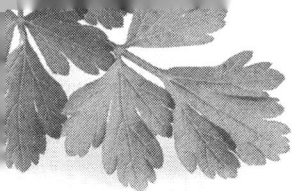

Cheddar Cheese and Bacon Risotto with Beer

(Prep Time: 15 MIN | Cook Time: 30 MIN | Serves: 8)

Ingredients:

For cooking:
1 tbsp low-calorie butter

For risotto:
½ yellow onion (peeled, finely chopped)

2 cloves garlic (peeled, minced)

2 cups Arborio rice

1 (12 ounce) bottle beer of choice

6 cups fat-free chicken stock

4 rashers extra lean turkey bacon (cooked, finely chopped)

1½ ounces Parmesan cheese (finely grated)

⅔ cup low-fat Cheddar cheese (shredded)

¼ tsp cayenne pepper

Directions:

1. In a large pan over moderately high heat, melt the butter.
2. Add the onion to the pan and sauté for 3-4 minutes. Add the minced garlic and cook for another 60 seconds.
3. Add the Arborio rice and cook, while stirring, for 2-3 minutes.
4. Pour in the beer and increase the temperature to high.
5. As the beer starts to simmer, turn the heat down to moderately low and pour in just half a cup of the chicken stock.
6. As soon as the stock has been absorbed, pour in another half a cup. Repeat this process until all of the stock has been used, the mixture is creamy, and the rice is al dente.
7. Take off the heat and sprinkle with the cooked bacon, cheeses, and cayenne pepper. Stir well until the cheeses melt into the risotto.
8. Serve.

Freestyle Smart Points Per Serving: 10

(Calories 280 | Total Fats 7g | Net Carbs: 41g | Protein 10g | Fiber: 0g)

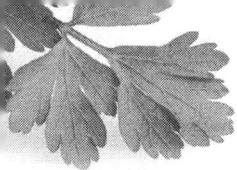

Chicken Lasagna

(Prep Time: 30 MIN | Cook Time: 1 HOUR 10 MIN | Serves: 10)

Ingredients:

For cooking:

Nonstick spray

For lasagna:

2 (25 ounce) jars marinara
sauce

1 (8 ounce) package no-boil
lasagne noodles

15 ounces fresh low-fat
ricotta cheese

2¼ cups low-fat mozzarella
cheese (shredded)

3 cups cooked rotisserie
chicken (chopped)

Directions:

1. Preheat the main oven to 375 degrees F. Spritz a 9x13" casserole dish with nonstick spray.

2. First, spread around 1 cup of marinara sauce in the base of the dish. Top with a third of the noodles in one single layer. Follow, by spreading all of the ricotta cheese evenly over the top of the noodles.

3. On top of the ricotta cheese, scatter 1 cup of mozzarella cheese, 1½ cups of the chopped chicken and another cup of marinara sauce.

4. Arrange the second third of the noodles in a single layer, top with the remaining chicken and another cup of shredded cheese.

5. Finish with a layer of noodles and pour over any remaining marinara sauce.

6. Cover the baking dish with aluminum foil and bake in the preheated oven for 60 minutes.

7. Remove the foil and top with the remaining shredded cheese. Return to the oven for another several minutes, or until the cheese is totally melted.

8. Remove the dish from the oven and set aside to rest 5-7 minutes.

9. Slice into ten even portions and serve.

Freestyle Smart Points Per Serving: 7

(Calories 350 | Total Fats 10g | Net Carbs: 32g | Protein 27g | Fiber: 4g)Bottom of Form

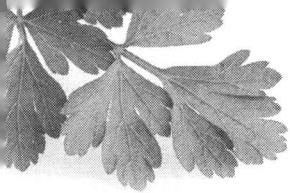

Creamy Pasta Salad with Avocado and Bacon

(Prep Time: 10 MIN | Cook Time: N/A | Serves: 8)

Ingredients:

For pasta salad:

4 cups cooked pasta
(preferably corkscrew-shaped)
8 rashers cooked centre-cut
bacon (diced)
1 cup cherry tomatoes
(quartered)
2 cups romaine lettuce
(shredded)

For dressing:

1 ripe, medium avocado
(peeled, pitted, mashed)
1½ tsp freshly squeezed lemon
juice
¼ cup low-fat mayo
1½ tsp apple cider vinegar
¼ tsp kosher salt
¼ tsp powdered garlic

Directions:

1. Add the pasta salad ingredients to a serving bowl, toss to combine and set to one side for a moment.
2. In a smaller bowl, add all of the dressing ingredients and whisk with a fork until smooth and combined.
3. Pour the dressing over the cooked pasta, gently toss until coated.
4. Keep chilled until ready to serve, enjoy at room temperature.

Freestyle Smart Points Per Serving: 5

(Calories 175 | Total Fats 6g | Net Carbs: 22g | Protein 6g | Fiber: 3g)

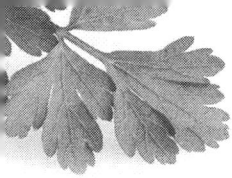

Hot 'n Creamy Chicken Penne

(Prep Time: 10 MIN | Cook Time: 35 MIN | Serves: 8)

Ingredients:

For cooking:

Nonstick spray

For pasta:

12 ounces penne pasta

2 cup chicken (shredded)

8 ounces fat-free cream cheese

½ cup hot sauce

1 (1 ounce) package ranch seasoning mix

½ cup fat-free sour cream

½ cup low-fat Cheddar cheese

For topping

½ cup low-fat sharp Cheddar cheese

Directions:

1. Preheat the main oven to 375 degrees F. Using nonstick spray, lightly spritz a 9x13" casserole dish and set to one side.
2. Cook the pasta according to the package directions, drain.
3. Combine the drained, cooked penne with the remaining pasta ingredients stirring gently until well combined. Transfer to a casserole dish and evenly spread.
4. Scatter the sharp Cheddar over the top and bake in the preheated oven for just under 20 minutes, or until the cheese melts.

Freestyle Smart Points Per Serving: 6

(Calories 270 | Total Fats 10g | Net Carbs: 18.5g | Protein 20.5g | Fiber: 2g)Bottom of Form

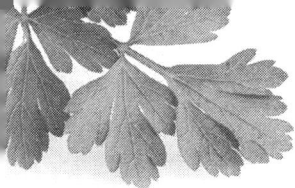

Mushroom and Garlic Quinoa

(Prep Time: 5 MIN | Cook Time: 5 HOUR 15 MIN | Serves: 6)

Ingredients:

For quinoa:

4 cups vegetable broth

2 cups quinoa (uncooked)

4 green onions (chopped)

12 ounces mushrooms (sliced)

4 ounces low-fat cream cheese

4 cloves garlic (peeled, minced)

1 tsp Italian seasoning

1½ tsp sea salt

1 tsp black pepper

½ cup Parmesan cheese (freshly grated**)**

Directions:

1. Add all of the ingredients, apart from the freshly grated Parmesan cheese to your slow cooker. Stir to combine.
2. On low heat, cook for 4-5 hours, until the quinoa is cooked through.
3. Scatter with the Parmesan and close the lid of the slow cooker, cook for another 15 minutes, until the cheese is totally melted.

Freestyle Smart Points Per Serving: 8

(Calories 310 | Total Fats 9g | Net Carbs: 39g | Protein 15g | Fiber: 5g) Bottom of Form

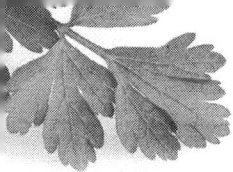

Pea and Scallop Linguine

(Prep Time: 10 MIN | Cook Time: 15 MIN | Serves: 2)

Ingredients:

For cooking:
1 tbsp salted butter

For pasta:
4 ounces whole wheat linguine

1 cup frozen petit pois

2 tbsp fresh parsley (chopped)

1 tsp good-quality olive oil

Sea salt and black pepper

6 large fresh scallops

Directions:

1. Cook the linguine in a deep pot of salted water according to packet directions. Four minutes before the pasta is due to finish cooking, add the petit pois to the water.

2. Drain the pasta and peas, reserving half a cup of the cooking liquid. Return the drained pasta to the pot along with the reserved cooking liquid, parsley, and olive oil. Taste and season with sea salt and black pepper as necessary.

3. While the pasta cooks, prepare the scallops.

4. Melt the butter in a skillet over moderate heat. Add the scallops and cook for 2 and a half minutes on one side, before flipping and cooking for another 40-50 seconds on the other side. The scallops should be opaque throughout.

5. Divide the cooked pasta between two bowls and top each with an equal amount of scallops. Serve straight away.

Freestyle Smart Points Per Serving: 7

(Calories 375 | Total Fats 7g | Net Carbs: 47g | Protein 27g | Fiber: 9g)

INSTANT POT
PASTA & GRAIN DISHES

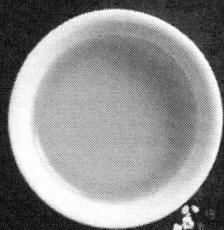

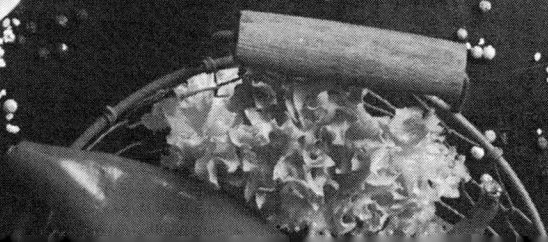

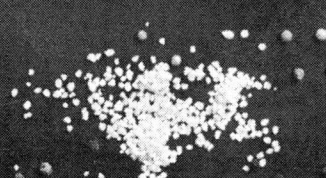

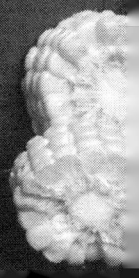

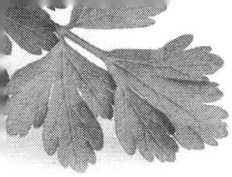

Cheesy Rigatoni

(Prep Time: 10 MIN | Cook Time: 17 MIN | Serves: 7)

Ingredients:

For cooking:
1 tsp butter

For rigatoni:
10 oz rigatoni pasta

8 oz broccoli, chopped

1 cup cheddar cheese, grated

½ cup heavy cream

1 cup tomatoes, diced

1 small onion, diced

1 tsp fresh lemon juice

Seasoning:
½ tsp dried oregano, ground

1 tsp sugar

1 tsp Italian seasoning

½ tsp red pepper flakes

Salt

Directions:

6. Place the pasta in the stainless steel insert of your Instant Pot. Sprinkle with some salt and securely lock the lid. Set the steam release handle and press the Manual button. Set the timer for 7 minutes and cook on High pressure.

7. When done, perform a quick pressure release and open the pot. Using a large colander, drain the pasta and remove the water.

8. Press the Sauté button and add butter. Gently stir until butter has completely melted. Add broccoli, onions, and heavy cream. Bring it to a boil and simmer for 3-4 minutes.

9. Add tomatoes, lemon juice, sugar, oregano, Italian seasoning, and red pepper flakes. Stir well and simmer for 6-7 minutes.

10. Finally, add pasta and give it a good stir.

11. Optionally, garnish with some fresh basil leaves and serve immediately.

Freestyle SmartPoints Per Serving: 7

(Calories 216 | Total Fats 10g | Net Carbs: 22.6g | Protein 8.8g | Fiber: 0g)

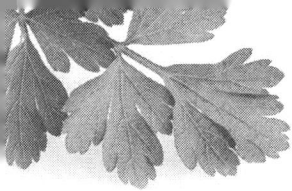

Quick Spicy Couscous

(Prep Time: 5 MIN | Cook Time: 3 MIN | Serves: 5)

Ingredients:

For cooking:

1 tsp olive oil

4 cups chicken broth, reduced sodium

For couscous:

2 cups couscous

1 small onion, diced

1 small carrot, diced

¼ cup fresh parsley, finely chopped

Seasoning:

½ tsp chili powder

¼ tsp garlic powder

½ tsp sea salt

¼ tsp black pepper, ground

Directions:

1. Place the butter in your Instant Pot. Press the Sauté button and gently stir until the butter has completely melted.
2. Add onions and sprinkle with garlic powder. Cook for 2-3 minutes, or until soft.
3. Add couscous and carrot. Sprinkle with chili powder, salt, and pepper. Stir well and pour in the chicken stock.
4. Securely lock the lid and adjust the steam release handle. Press the Manual button and set the timer for 3 minutes. Cook on High pressure.
5. When you hear the cooker's end signal, perform a quick pressure release by moving the valve to the Venting position.
6. Open the pot and stir in the parsley. Transfer to a serving dish and serve immediately. Enjoy!

Freestyle SmartPoints Per Serving: 8

(Calories 310 | Total Fats 2.5g | Net Carbs: 52.7g | Protein 13g | Fiber: 4.1g)

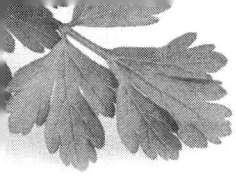

Avocado Ziti with Cheese

(Prep Time: 10 MIN | Cook Time: 13 MIN | Serves: 6)

Ingredients:

For cooking:
1 tsp olive oil

Water

For avocado ziti:
½ ripe avocado, cut into cubes

10 oz ziti pasta

1 small red onion, chopped

1 cup button mushrooms, sliced

¼ cup sour cream, low-fat

1 tbsp Parmesan cheese, grated

Seasoning:
1 tsp fresh rosemary, finely chopped

½ tsp dried thyme, ground

Salt

Black pepper

Directions:

1. Plug in the Instant Pot and place the pasta in the stainless steel insert. Pour in 3 cups of water and sprinkle with some salt. Close the lid and adjust the steam release handle. Press the Manual button and set the timer for 6 minutes. Cook on High pressure.

2. When you hear the cooker's end signal, perform a quick pressure release and open the pot. Using a large colander, drain the pasta and remove the liquid. Place in a large bowl and set aside.

3. Heat up the olive oil in the inner pot over the Sauté mode. Add mushrooms and cook for 5 minutes, or until soften. Add onions and heavy cream. Stir well and bring it to a boil.

4. Finally, add avocado cubes and sprinkle with thyme, rosemary, salt, and pepper. Cook for 3-4 minutes more, stirring occasionally. Turn off the pot and transfer all to a bowl with pasta. Give it a good stir and transfer to a serving plate. Sprinkle with Parmesan cheese before serving. Enjoy!

Freestyle SmartPoints Per Serving: 6

(Calories 212 | Total Fats 7.7g | Net Carbs: 27.8g | Protein 7.2g | Fiber: 1.5g)

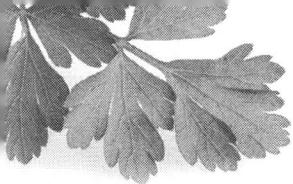

Zucchini Farfalline

(Prep Time: 10 MIN | Cook Time: 18 MIN | Serves: 7)

Ingredients:

For cooking:

1 tsp olive oil

1 cup vegetable broth

Water

Seasoning:

1 tsp Italian seasoning

½ tsp dried oregano, ground

½ tsp sea salt

½ tsp red pepper

For zucchini farfalline:

1 medium-sized zucchini, chopped

1 lb farfalline pasta

1 medium-sized parsnip, chopped

1 cup cherry tomatoes, halved

1 small onion, chopped

2 garlic cloves, finely chopped

1 tbsp fresh parsley, finely chopped

1 tsp soy sauce

Directions:

1. Plug in the Instant Pot and add oil to the stainless steel insert. Heat over the Sauté button and add onions and garlic. Cook for 3-4 minutes, or until translucent.
2. Add zucchini, parsnip, and parsley. Sprinkle with Italian seasoning, oregano, salt, and pepper. Stir well and cook for 2-4 minutes more. Stir in the tomatoes and vegetable broth. Bring it to a boil and cook for 5 minutes, stirring occasionally.
3. Remove all to a large bowl and cover with a lid.
4. Now, pour 3 cups of water in the inner pot. Add pasta and sprinkle with some salt. Securely lock the lid and adjust the steam release handle. Press the Manual button and set the timer for 6 minutes. Cook on High pressure.
5. When you hear the cooker's end signal, perform a quick pressure release and open the pot.
6. Mix pasta with zucchini mixture and transfer to a serving plate. Garnish with some cucumber slices and serve immediately.

Freestyle SmartPoints Per Serving: 5

(Calories 223 | Total Fats 2.5g | Net Carbs: 39.8g | Protein 8.7g | Fiber: 1.5g)

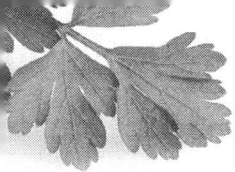

Cajun Chicken Risotto

(Prep Time: 15 MIN | Cook Time: 20 MIN | Serves:)

Ingredients:

For cooking:
1 tsp olive oil

Water

For risotto:
½ cup rice

7 oz chicken breasts, skinless, boneless, and chopped into bite-sized pieces

2 slices of bacon, chopped

1 medium-sized tomato, chopped

1 red bell pepper, sliced

¼ cup green peas

1 tbsp celery stalks, finely chopped

Seasoning:
2 tsp Cajun seasoning

½ tsp white pepper

2 tsp turmeric powder

Salt

Directions:

1. Place the chicken in a deep bowl and sprinkle with Cajun seasoning and white pepper. Let it sit for 20-25 minutes.

2. Plug in the Instant Pot and place the rice in the stainless steel insert. Add ½ cup of water and sprinkle with some salt. Securely lock the lid and adjust the steam release handle. Press the Manual button and set the timer for 4 minutes. Cook on High pressure.

3. When done, perform a quick pressure release and open the pot. Transfer the rice to a bowl and add turmeric powder. Stir until well combined and set aside. Clean the pot.

4. Now, press the Sauté button and add bacon. Cook for 3-4 minutes, or until crisp. Remove the bacon to a small plate and set aside.

5. Grease the inner pot with olive oil and add chicken. Cook for 5 minutes, or until golden brown. Add tomato, celery, bell pepper, and green peas. Bring it to a boil and cook for additional 3-4 minutes. Turn off the pot and transfer all to a large bowl. Add rice and give it a good stir.

6. Optionally, sprinkle with some finely chopped cilantro before serving. Enjoy!

Freestyle SmartPoints Per Serving: 5

(Calories 210 | Total Fats 7.3g | Net Carbs: 17.5g | Protein 16.5g | Fiber: 1.3g)

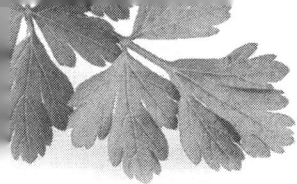

Shrimp Linguine

(Prep Time: 5 MIN | Cook Time: 15 MIN | Serves: 8)

Ingredients:

For cooking:
1 tsp butter
Water

For shrimps:
12 oz shrimps, peeled and deveined
1 small red onion, diced
2 garlic cloves, minced
1 tbsp dry sherry
½ tsp balsamic vinegar
1/3 cup heavy cream
1 tbsp cheddar cheese
½ tsp cayenne pepper
Salt
Pepper

For linguine pasta:
12 oz linguine pasta
½ tsp dried thyme, ground
½ tsp dried rosemary, ground
Salt

Directions:

1. Plug in the Instant Pot and place the pasta in the stainless steel insert. Add 4 cups of water and sprinkle with some salt. Close the lid and set the steam release handle. Press the Manual button and set the timer for 7 minutes. Cook on High pressure.

2. When done, perform a quick pressure release and open the pot. Drain the pasta and place in a large bowl. Sprinkle with thyme and rosemary and give it a good stir. Set aside.

3. Now, melt the butter in the inner pot over the Sauté button. Add shrimps and sprinkle with cayenne pepper, salt, and pepper. Cook for 2 minutes on each side. Transfer the shrimps to a bowl with pasta cover with a lid.

4. Add onions, garlic, and dry sherry to the pot. Stir-fry for 4-5 minutes or until the onions translucent.

5. Stir in the heavy cream and balsamic vinegar. Bring it to a boil and simmer for 2-3 minutes more.

6. Pour the sauce over shrimps and pasta. Give it a good stir and serve immediately.

Freestyle SmartPoints Per Serving: 5

(Calories 204 | Total Fats 4.4g | Net Carbs: 25g | Protein 15g | Fiber: 0.3g)

SOUPS, STEWS, CHILIES

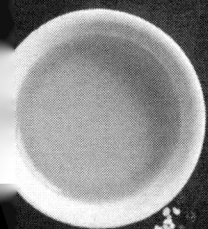

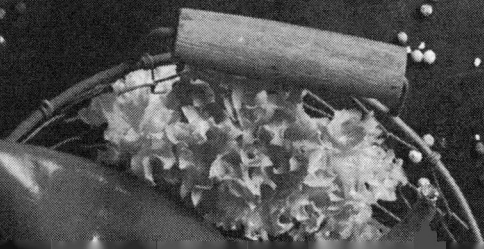

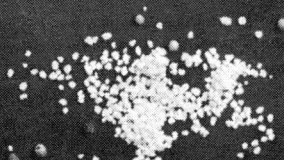

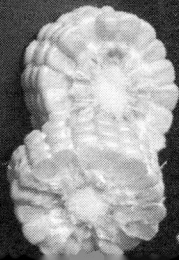

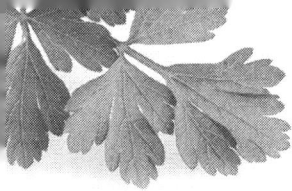

Green Chile Chicken

(Prep Time: 5 MIN | Cook Time: 7 HOUR 30 MIN | Serves: 11)

Ingredients:

For chilli:

2 pounds chicken breast
(uncooked)
2 (15 ½ ounce) cans navy
beans (drained)
2 (4 ounce) cans mild green
chilies (diced)
2 ½ cups corn (frozen)
1 ¾ cups low-salt chicken
broth
½ cup half and half
4 ounces light cream cheese

For seasoning:

1 tsp black pepper
2 tsp cumin
2 tsp onion powder
1 tsp sea salt
2 tsp powdered garlic
¼ tsp cayenne pepper
2 tsp chili powder
1 tsp seasoned salt

Directions:

1. Add the chicken, navy beans, chilies, corn, chicken broth, and seasoning to a slow cooker. Cover and on low, cook for between 7 hours.

2. Remove the chicken and, using two metal forks, shred the meat. Stir the chicken back into the chili and add, while stirring the half and half, followed by the cream cheese. Cook for half an hour, on high. Serve in bowls.

Freestyle SmartPoints Per Serving: 2

(Calories 229 | Total Fats 4.5g | Net Carbs: 14.5g | Protein 25g | Fiber: 3.5g)Bottom of Form

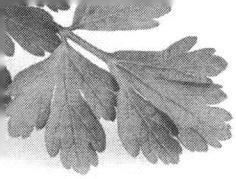

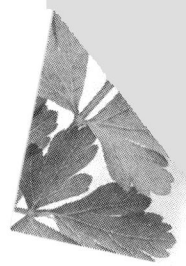

Hot Thai Squash Soup

(Prep Time: 15 MIN | Cook Time: 4 HOUR | Serves: 4)

Ingredients:

For soup:

2 pounds butternut squash (peeled, cut into 1 inch chunks)

2 cups low-salt, fat-free chicken broth

2 cups unsweetened coconut milk (carton, not canned)

¼ cup onion (peeled, chopped)

1 tbsp packed brown sugar

1 tbsp sriracha hot sauce

1 tbsp soy sauce

2 tbsp freshly squeezed lime juice

For topping:

1 tbsp lime zest

¼ cup fresh basil (chopped)

¼ cup peanuts (chopped)

Directions:

1. In a slow cooker, add all of the soup ingredients. Cover and cook for 4 hours on Low.
2. As soon as the soup is sufficiently cooked, blend the ingredients until smooth.
3. In a large dish, combine the topping ingredients.
4. Serve the soup with 2 tablespoons of topping.

Freestyle SmartPoints Per Serving: 4

(Calories 202 | Total Fats 7g | Net Carbs: 28g | Protein 5g | Fiber: 6g)Bottom of Form

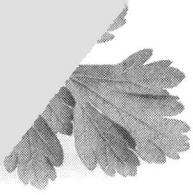

Lasagna Noodle Soup

(Prep Time: 5 MIN | Cook Time 6 HOUR 30 MIN | Serves: 8)

Ingredients:

For soup:

1 pound vegetarian crumbles

1 onion (peeled, diced)

6 cloves garlic (peeled, minced)

1 (28 ounce) can crushed tomatoes

1 (16 ounce) jar sugar-free marinara sauce

3 cups vegetable broth

2 tsp Italian seasoning

10 whole wheat lasagne noodles

1 medium zucchini (roughly chopped)

6 ounces fresh spinach

½ cup Parmesan cheese

Sea salt and black pepper

Directions:

1. Add the vegetarian crumble, onion, garlic, tomatoes, marinara sauce, vegetable broth and Italian seasoning to a slow cooker.
2. Cook for 6 hours on a low heat.
3. Open the cooker and add the lasagna noodles, followed by the zucchini, and spinach. Cook for another half an hour, until the noodles are al dente.
4. Stir in the cheese, season and enjoy.

Freestyle SmartPoints Per Serving: 6

(Calories 313 | Total Fats 5g | Net Carbs: 39g | Protein 25g | Fiber: 11g)Bottom of Form

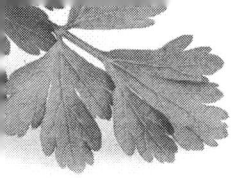

Oriental Wonton Soup

(Prep Time: 3 MIN | Cook Time: 5 MIN | Serves: 4)

Ingredients:

For soup:

6 cups low-salt chicken broth

¼ cup low-salt soy sauce

3 tbsp rice wine vinegar

1 tbsp ginger (minced)

1 tbsp sesame oil

16 frozen, store-bought dumplings (any brand)

2 cups mushrooms (sliced)

4 cups baby spinach

8 ounces rice noodles (cooked, to serve)

Cilantro (garnish)

Directions:

1. In a pot, bring the broth, soy sauce, vinegar, ginger, and sesame oil to the boil, whisking occasionally.

2. Add the dumplings, followed by the mushrooms and spinach and simmer for 2-3 minutes, or until the dumplings are warm and the kale wilts.

3. Cook the noodles according to the package instructions and evenly divide between 4 bowls.

4. Ladle equal amounts of wonton soup over the noodles and garnish with cilantro.

Freestyle SmartPoints Per Serving: 4

(Calories 325 | Total Fats 4g | Net Carbs: 12.5g | Protein 12g | Fiber: 7g)Bottom of Form

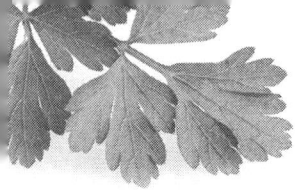

Squash Stuffed with Turkey Chili

(Prep Time: 5 MIN | Cook Time: 1 HOUR 30 MIN | Serves: 4)

Ingredients:

For cooking:

Nonstick spray

For seasoning:

¾ tsp cumin

¼ tsp chili powder

¼ tsp paprika

1 bay leaf

For chili:

2 acorn squash (seeded, halved)

1 pound 95% lean ground turkey

½ tsp sea salt

1 red onion (peeled, chopped)

2 garlic cloves (peeled, crushed)

1 (10 ounce) can mild tomatoes with green chilies

½ cup canned tomato sauce

½ cup cold water

6 tbsp sharp Cheddar cheese (freshly grated)

Cilantro (chopped, to garnish)

Directions:

1. Preheat the main oven to 400 degrees F. Spritz a baking tray with nonstick spray.
2. Arrange the squash on the tray, cut sides facing downwards, and bake in the oven until soft, between 30-35 minutes.
3. In the meantime, in a large frying pan, brown the turkey over moderately high heat, using the back of a wooden spoon to break the meat up as it cooks. Season with salt.
4. When the turkey is sufficiently cooked through, add the onion, followed by the garlic, and cook for a few minutes over moderate heat.
5. Add the can of tomatoes, along with the tomato sauce, water, and seasoning.
6. Cover with a lid and simmer for 20-25 minutes over moderately low heat, stirring occasionally.
7. Remove and discard the bay leaf, turn the squash over and fill each half with chili, around ¾ cup in quantity is perfect.
8. Scatter with cheese and bake for 5 minutes, until the cheese is melted.
9. Garnish with cilantro and serve.

Freestyle SmartPoints Per Serving: 5

(Calories 320 | Total Fats 12g | Net Carbs: 24.5g | Protein 28g | Fiber: 5g)

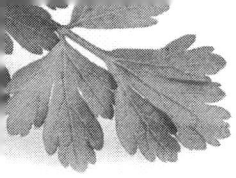

Cajun Soup

(Prep Time: 20 MIN | Cook Time: 6 HOUR 10 MIN | Serves: 14)

Ingredients:

For cooking:
2 tsp virgin olive oil

For soup:
1 medium onion (peeled, chopped)

2 stalks celery (chopped)

1 green bell pepper (chopped)

2 cloves garlic (peeled, minced)

6 ounces chicken andouille (chopped)

8 ounces lean ham (cubed)

1 (28-ounce) can fire roasted diced tomatoes

3 cups water

3 cups chicken broth

2 tsp Cajun seasoning

16 ounces frozen corn kernels

Seasoning:
Sea salt and black pepper

Directions:

1. In a skillet over moderate heat, heat the oil. Add the onion followed by the celery and pepper and cook, while stirring for 5-7 minutes, until softened. Add the garlic and cook, continually stirring for 60 seconds.
2. Transfer the mixture to a 5-6 quart slow cooker and add all remaining soup ingredients.
3. Cover, and on low heat, cook for between 4-6 hours, until the vegetables are fork tender.
4. Taste and season as necessary.

Freestyle Smart Points Per Serving: 2

(Calories 91 | Total Fats 2.5g | Net Carbs: 8.5g | Protein 8g | Fiber: 2g)

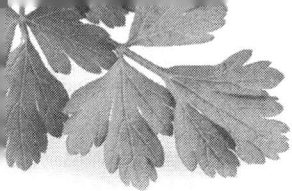

Cauliflower Cheese Soup with Bacon

(Prep Time: 15 MIN | Cook Time: 20 MIN | Serves: 5)

Ingredients:

For soup:

6 cups cauliflower (cut into florets)

2 ribs celery

½ onion (peeled)

2 cloves garlic (peeled)

8 slices turkey bacon (chopped)

2 cups vegetable broth

2 cups non-fat milk

2 tbsp flour

2 tbsp water

Salt and black pepper

1½ cups low-fat Cheddar cheese (shredded)

3 scallions (diced, for garnish)

Seasoning:

Sea salt and black pepper

Cayenne pepper

Directions:

1. Add the cauliflower florets to a food processor and on the pulse setting, process until finely chopped.
2. Remove the chopped cauliflower and set to one side.
3. Add the celery, onion, and garlic to the food processor and pulse once more until finely chopped.
4. To a large pan, add the turkey bacon, cooking until crisp. Remove the bacon and set to one side. Drain away all but 1 tbsp of the bacon drippings from the pan.
5. Add the chopped onion mixture to the pan and cook until fragrant, for approximately 2-3 minutes.
6. Next, add the cauliflower and pour in the vegetable broth and milk. Bring to a boil before reducing to a simmer. Continue simmering for 7-10 minutes or until the cauliflower is fork tender.
7. Combine the flour with the water and add the mixture to the soup. Bring to a boil, before reducing to simmer for a couple of minutes; this will help to thicken the soup. Taste and season as necessary.
8. Remove the soup from the heat and add the cheese and bacon, stirring thoroughly to combine.
9. Serve garnished with scallions.

Freestyle Smart Points Per Serving: 6

(Calories 224 | Total Fats 6g | Net Carbs: 13g | Protein 18g | Fiber: 3g)

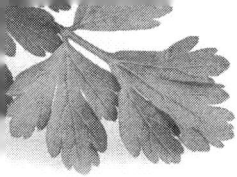

Coconut Curry and Tomato Chickpea Soup

(Prep Time: 5 MIN | Cook Time: 45 MIN | Serves: 4)

Ingredients:

For cooking:
2 tsp coconut oil

For bake:
1 onion (peeled, diced)

1 tbsp curry powder

1 bay leaf

4 garlic cloves (peeled, minced)

1 tbsp ginger (minced)

1 cup potatoes (chopped)

1 (28-ounce) can crushed tomatoes

1 cup canned light coconut milk

1 cup vegetable broth

1 (14-ounce) can chickpeas (drained, rinsed)

4 cups kale (chopped)

3 cups cauliflower florets

Seasoning:
Sea salt and black pepper

Directions:

1. Over moderate heat, heat the coconut oil. Add the onions and cook until completely softened, for approximately 5-7 minutes. Add the curry powder followed by the bay leaf and cook for a few more minutes. Add the garlic and ginger, and cook for 60 seconds.

2. Add the potatoes along with the canned tomatoes. Pour in the coconut milk and vegetable broth and bring to the boil. Cover with a tight-fitting lid, and simmer until the potatoes are fork-tender, this will take 20-25 minutes.

3. Add the rinsed chickpeas, chopped kale, and florets. Cook for 10-15 minutes, until the cauliflower florets are fork-tender and the kale is beginning to wilt.

4. Season to taste and serve.

Freestyle Smart Points Per Serving: 4

(Calories 369 | Total Fats 10g | Net Carbs: 52g | Protein 16g | Fiber: 8g)

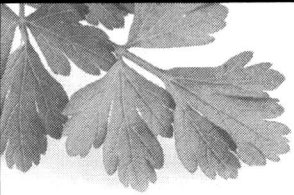

Fiery Fajita Chicken Soup

(Prep Time: 10 MIN | Cook Time: 6 HOURS | Serves: 6)

Ingredients:

For soup:

2 tbsp olive oil

2 pounds skinless, boneless chicken thighs

32 ounces low sodium chicken broth

1 (14-ounce) can fire roasted diced tomatoes

2 green peppers (seeded, diced)

2 red peppers (seeded, diced)

1 onion (peeled, thinly sliced)

2 cups mushrooms (halved)

3 cloves garlic (peeled, minced)

1 jalapeno (seeded, minced)

Seasoning:

2 tsp cumin

1½ tsp chili powder

1 tsp paprika

1 tsp oregano

½ tsp coriander

Sea salt and black pepper

Directions:

1. Add all the soup ingredients to a slow cooker, stir well and then add the seasoning. On low heat, cook for 6 hours.

2. Using 2 forks; shred the chicken.

3. Serve hot.

Freestyle Smart Points Per Serving: 5

(Calories 305 | Total Fats 11g | Net Carbs: 11g | Protein 34g | Fiber: 3g)

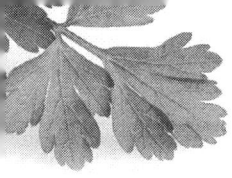

New England Clam Chowder

(Prep Time: 10 MIN | Cook Time: 8 HOUR 5 MIN | Serves: 6)

Ingredients:

For soup:

2 (6½ ounce) cans chopped clams

2 cups waxy potatoes (peeled, cut into ½" pieces)

1 cup yellow onion (peeled, chopped)

1 cup celery with leaves (chopped)

½ cup green bell pepper (chopped)

1 (14-ounce) can Italian-style stewed tomatoes (undrained)

1½ cups spicy tomato juice

½ tsp sea salt

1 tsp dried thyme (crushed)

1 bay leaf

For serving:

¼ cup fresh parsley (chopped)

4 slices cooked, crispy bacon (drained, crumbled)

Directions:

1. First, drain the clam liquid from the cans into a 3½-4 quart slow cooker. Transfer the clams themselves to a re-sealable container and chill until ready to use.
2. Add all remaining soup ingredients to the clam liquid in the slow cooker.
3. Cover, and on low, cook for between 6-8 hours, until the veggies are fork-tender.
4. Add the chilled chopped clams and increase the slow cooker to a high heat setting. Cover and cook for 5 minutes, or until the clams are heated through. Discard the bay leaf.
5. Garnish with fresh parsley and crumbled, crispy bacon and serve.

Freestyle Smart Points Per Serving: 2

(Calories 106 | Total Fats 2.5g | Net Carbs: 17g | Protein 6g | Fiber: 3g)

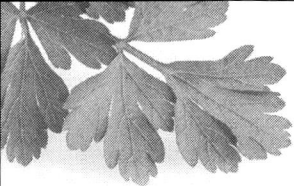

Pea and Ham Soup

(Prep Time: 10 MIN | Cook Time: 8 HOUR | Serves: 6)

Ingredients:

For soup:

2¼ cups dried split peas
(rinsed, drained)

1 leftover ham bone

2 carrots (peeled, chopped)

2 stalks celery (chopped)

1 medium onion (peeled,
chopped)

4 cups fat-free chicken broth

4 cups water

2 bay leaves

1 tsp dried thyme

1 cup cooked ham (diced)

Directions:

1. Add all of the soup ingredients, excluding the cooked ham to a 5-6 quart slow cooker and stir well.

2. Cover, and on low, cook for between 6-8 hours, until the peas are fork-tender.

3. Discard the ham bone and bay leaves.

4. Stir in the cooked, diced ham and serve.

Freestyle Smart Points Per Serving: 2

(Calories 271 | Total Fats 2g | Net Carbs: 26g | Protein 21g | Fiber: 17.5g)

Three-Bean Hot Turkey Sausage Chili

(Prep Time: 15 MIN | Cook Time: 8 HOUR 10 MIN | Serves: 10)

Ingredients:

Toppings:

1 red onion (peeled, chopped)

Fresh cilantro (chopped)

Low-fat Cheddar cheese (shredded)

For chili:

1 pound Italian style hot turkey sausage

1 cup onion (peeled, chopped)

1 (28 ounce) can diced tomatoes

1 (14 ounce) can tomato sauce

1 (6 ounce) can chopped green chiles (drained)

1 (14 ounce) can chickpeas (rinsed, drained)

1 (14 ounce) can black beans (rinsed, drained)

1 (14 ounce) can pinto beans (rinsed, drained)

1½ tbsp chili powder

1½ tsp ground cumin

1 tsp garlic powder

1 tsp dried oregano

Directions:

1. Using a microwave, cook the turkey and onion (in a microwave-safe bowl) for 5-7 minutes, until the onions are soft, and the turkey meat is no longer pink.
2. Drain away any excess fat and transfer the mixture to a slow cooker along with all remaining chili ingredients.
3. Cover and on low, cook for between 6-8 hours.
4. Top with chopped onion, cilantro, and shredded cheese. Serve,

Freestyle Smart Points Per Serving: 2

(Calories 213 | Total Fats 6g | Net Carbs: 19g | Protein 15g | Fiber:7g)

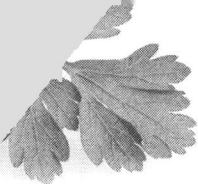

White Bean Leftover Turkey Chili

(Prep Time: 15 MIN | Cook Time: 1 HOUR 15 MIN | Serves: 8)

Ingredients:

For cooking:

2 tbsp olive oil

For chili:

½ cup yellow onion (peeled, diced)

½ green bell pepper (diced)

½ cup celery (diced)

1 tbsp garlic (peeled, minced)

2 cups chicken broth

3 (15 ounce) cans white beans

2 cups leftover cooked turkey (shredded)

Seasoning:

¼ tsp cayenne pepper

1 tsp ground cumin

¾ tsp oregano

½ tsp sea salt

¼ tsp freshly ground black pepper

Directions:

1. Heat the oil in a deep pot, add the onion, followed by the green pepper, and celery. Cook over moderately high heat until the onions are softened and translucent and the green peppers fork tender. Stir in the minced garlic.

2. Pour in the broth, and add the white beans, and shredded turkey, stirring well.

3. Add the seasonings and stir to combine. Bring to a boil and then reduce to a simmer. Cover for 30-60 minutes, occasionally stirring.

4. Serve.

Freestyle Smart Points Per Serving: 1

(Calories 462 | Total Fats 5.5g | Net Carbs: 40g | Protein 44.5g | Fiber: 19g)

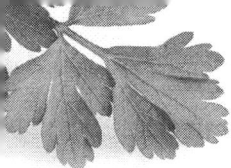

Fiery Caribbean Chicken Stew

(Prep Time: 20 MIN | Cook Time: 35 MIN | Serves: 6)

Ingredients:

For cooking:

1 tsp coconut oil

For chicken:

1 fresh lime

6 chicken thighs (skin removed)

6 chicken drumsticks (skin removed)

1 medium carrot (finely chopped)

2 tsp cornstarch

1½ cups unsweetened light coconut milk

¼ tsp sea salt

For marinade:

1 large tomato (chopped)

4 medium scallions (chopped)

1 large onion (peeled, chopped)

2 cloves garlic (peeled, chopped)

¾ Scotch Bonnet pepper (seeded, membrane removed, chopped)

4 sprigs fresh thyme

2 tbsp low-salt soy sauce

Directions:

1. Squeeze the fresh lime over the chicken.
2. Using clean hands combine the marinade ingredients in a mixing bowl. Add the chicken to the bowl and allow to marinate for a minimum of 60 minutes.
3. Heat the oil in a saucepan over moderately high heat.
4. Take the chicken out of the marinade, reserving the marinade.
5. Add the chicken to the pan and sauté until browned all over.
6. Pour the marinade over the chicken and add the chopped carrots. Stir and cook for approximately 10 minutes.
7. Combine the cornstarch with the light coconut milk and pour into the pan. Continue to cook for 20 minutes.
8. Season to taste, and serve.

Freestyle Smart Points Per Serving: 6

(Calories 235 | Total Fats 9g | Net Carbs: 7g | Protein 27.5g | Fiber: 1.5g)

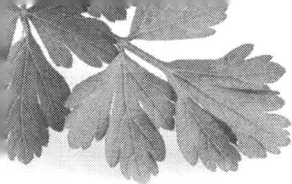

Mexican Chicken Tortilla Soup

(Prep Time: 20 MIN | Cook Time: 4 HOUR | Serves: 8)

Ingredients:

1 pound cooked chicken (shredded)

1 yellow onion (peeled, chopped)

1 (10 ounce) jar enchilada sauce

2 garlic cloves (peeled, minced)

1 (15 ounce) can chopped tomatoes

1 (4 ounce) can green chili peppers (finely chopped)

2 cups cold water

1 (14½ ounce) can chicken broth

10 ounces frozen corn

1 tbsp cilantro (chopped)

Seasoning:

1 tsp chili powder

1 tsp cumin

1 bay leaf

1 tsp sea salt

¼ tsp black pepper

For tortillas:

7 yellow corn tortillas

Canola oil

Directions:

1. Add the shredded chicken, onion, enchilada sauce, garlic, tomatoes, and chili pepper in your slow cooker. Pour in the water along with the chicken broth, and seasoning.
2. Stir in the frozen corn followed by the cilantro.
3. Cover with a tight-fitting lid, and on a low setting, cook for 3-4 hours, on high.
4. Preheat the main oven to 400 degrees F.
5. Lightly brush both sides of the tortillas with canola oil. Cut the tortilla into fine strips and arrange them, in a single layer, on a baking tray.
6. Bake in the oven for between 10-15 minutes, until crisp.
7. Scatter the crisp tortilla strips over the soup and serve.

Freestyle Smart Points Per Serving: 7

(Calories 262 | Total Fats 11g | Net Carbs: 21g | Protein 18g | Fiber: 4g)

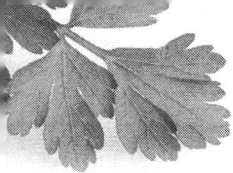

Mixed Vegetable and Lentil Stew

(Prep Time: 15 MIN | Cook Time: 8 HOUR 10 MIN | Serves: 6)

Ingredients:

For vegetables:

2 cups butternut squash (peeled, cubed)

2 cups red potatoes (chopped)

2 cups carrots (chopped)

1½ cups dry lentils

2 cups celery (chopped)

1 medium onion (peeled, diced)

4 garlic cloves (peeled, minced)

8 cups vegetable broth

2 tbsp virgin olive oil

4 cups spinach

½ cup parsley

Seasoning:

2 tsp herbs de Provence

1 tsp smoked paprika

1 tsp kosher salt

Salt and black pepper

Directions:

1. Add the butternut squash, potatoes, carrots, lentils, celery, onion, garlic, broth, and seasoning to a slow cooker, and on low heat, cook for between 7-8 hours.

2. Add approximately a third of the soup to a food blender together with the oil and process until lump free. Return to the slow cooker.

3. Stir in the spinach and parsley and cook for another 6-10 minutes, until the spinach begins to wilt.

Freestyle Smart Points Per Serving: 4

(Calories 320 | Total Fats 5g | Net Carbs: 36g | Protein 16g | Fiber: 19g)

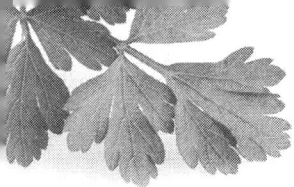

Salmon and Potato Chowder

(Prep Time: 20 MIN | Cook Time: 40 MIN | Serves: 6)

Ingredients:

For cooking:

1 tbsp olive oil

For chowder:

1 red or white onion (peeled, chopped)

1 celery stalk (diced)

½ red bell pepper (diced)

3 garlic cloves

2 tbsp fresh thyme (chopped)

½ tsp red pepper flakes

½ pound potatoes

2¾ cups vegetable broth

¾ cup frozen corn

¼ cup all-purpose flour

2½ cups skim milk

¾ tsp salt

½ tsp ground pepper

1¼ pounds fresh salmon (cut into 1" pieces)

¼ cup flat leaf parsley (minced)

Directions:

1. Over moderate heat, in a deep pot, add the oil.
2. Add the onion, followed by the celery, and bell pepper, and cook for 4-5 minutes.
3. Add the garlic along with the thyme, and red pepper flakes, and cook for 60 seconds.
4. Add the potatoes and pour in the vegetable broth. Bring to boil, before reducing the heat a little and simmering until the potatoes are fork tender, approximately 15 minutes.
5. Stir in the frozen corn and simmer for a couple of minutes.
6. In a mixing bowl, whisk the flour with the milk until lump free and add to the pan along with the salt and pepper. Cook, while whisking for several minutes until nice and thick.
7. Add the salmon and cook for another several minutes until the fish is cooked through.
8. Stir in the parsley and serve.

Freestyle Smart Points Per Serving: 4

(Calories 325 | Total Fats 11.5g | Net Carbs: 21.5g | Protein 31.5g | Fiber: 2.5g)

INSTANT POT SOUPS, STEWS AND CHILIES

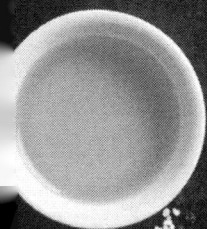

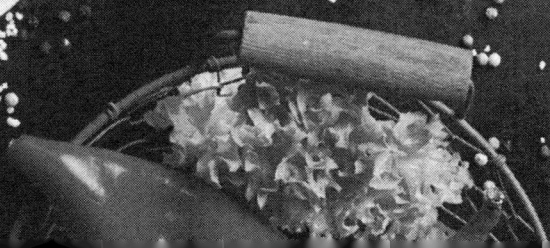

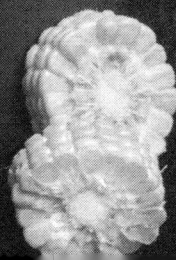

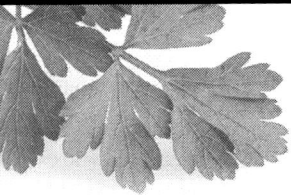

Green Chicken Curry

Ingredients:

For cooking:
1 tbsp oil

For curry:
7oz chicken breast

2 tbsp green curry paste

¾ cup coconut milk, reduced fat

½ cup green bell peppers, sliced

2 large onions, finely chopped

1 small tomato, sliced

¼ cup fish sauce

Seasoning:
1 tsp coconut sugar

1 tsp dried basil

Directions:

1. Grease the bottom of the inner pot with oil and heat up on the Sauté mode. Add the meat and briefly cook for 2-3 minutes, stirring constantly.
2. Now add green bell peppers, onions, and tomato. Cook for another 3-4 minutes, stirring constantly.
3. Pour in the coconut milk and 2 cups of water. Add green curry paste and bring it to a boil, stirring constantly.
4. Add the remaining ingredients and seal the lid. Set the steam release handle and cook for 20 minutes on the Manual mode.
5. When done, perform a quick pressure release and open the lid. Serve immediately.

Freestyle SmartPoints Per Serving: 5

(Calories 174 | Total Fats 11.4g | Net Carbs: 8g | Protein 9.1g | Fiber: 2g)

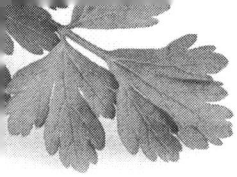

Pepper Chuck Roast Stew

(Prep Time: 15 MIN | Cook Time: 6 HOURS | Serves: 6)

Ingredients:

For cooking:

3 cups beef stock

For stew:

1 lb lean beef chuck roast, cut into bite-sized pieces

1 small red onion, sliced

1 cup baby potatoes, cut into cubes

1 large yellow bell pepper, chopped

2 tbsp fresh parsley, finely chopped

1 small celery stalk, chopped

Seasoning:

½ tsp smoked paprika, ground

½ tsp dried thyme, ground

¼ tsp chili powder

Salt

Black pepper

Directions:

1. Rinse the meat under cold running water and pat dry with a kitchen paper. Transfer to a cutting board and trim off any fat. Cut into bite-sized pieces.

2. Place the meat on the bottom of the stainless steel insert of your Instant Pot. Add vegetables and then sprinkle with paprika, thyme, salt, and pepper.

3. Pour in the beef stock and securely lock the lid. Set the steam release handle by moving the valve to the Sealing position.

4. Set the timer for 6 hours on Slow Cooker mode. Cook on High pressure.

5. When you hear the cooker's end signal, release the pressure naturally.

6. Open the pot and transfer into serving bowls. Sprinkle with fresh parsley and serve immediately.

7. Enjoy!

Freestyle SmartPoints Per Serving: 3

(Calories 165 | Total Fats 5.1g | Net Carbs: 2.9g | Protein 24.9g | Fiber: 0.8g)

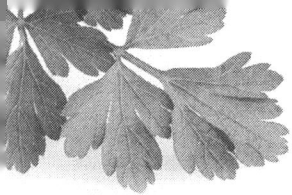

Green Bean Soup with Beef

(Prep Time: 15 MIN | Cook Time: 35 MIN | Serves: 6)

Ingredients:

For cooking:

2 cups beef broth

1 tsp olive oil

For soup:

1 lb green beans, chopped

6 oz lean beef tenderloin, cut into bite-sized pieces

1 small carrot, sliced

1 medium-sized red onion, chopped

2 cups cauliflower, chopped

1 tbsp fresh parsley, finely chopped

1 tbsp tomato paste

Seasoning:

¼ tsp dried thyme, ground

½ tsp dried basil, ground

1 tsp salt

½ tsp black pepper, ground

Directions:

1. Plug in the Instant Pot and add oil to the stainless steel insert. Press the Sauté button and heat. Add meat and cook for 5 minutes, or until browned.

2. Now, add green beans, carrot, onion, cauliflower, and parsley. Pour in the broth and add 2 cups of water. Stir in the thyme, basil, salt, and pepper.

3. Securely lock the lid and set the steam release handle by moving the valve to the Sealing position. Set the timer for 40 minutes and cook on High pressure.

4. When done, perform a quick pressure release and open the pot.

5. Stir in the tomato paste and continue to cook for 5 more minutes over Sauté mode.

6. For a creamy version, add ¼ cup of sour cream and bring it to a boil. Cook for additional 5 minutes. Enjoy!

Freestyle SmartPoints Per Serving: 2

(Calories 117 | Total Fats 3.2g | Net Carbs: 6.4g | Protein 12.7g | Fiber: 4.1g)

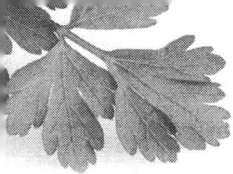

Lamb Parsnip Stew

(Prep Time: 15 MIN | Cook Time: 30 MIN | Serves: 5)

Ingredients:

For cooking:

2 cups beef broth

1 tsp butter, unsalted

Water

Seasoning:

½ tsp dried parsley, ground

½ tsp dried rosemary, ground

1 tsp cayenne pepper, ground

1 bay leaf

Salt

For stew:

1 lb leg of lamb, boneless and chopped

1 cup parsnips, chopped

2 cups tomatoes, diced

1 medium-sized carrot, sliced

1 medium-sized onion, chopped

1 cup baby potatoes, chopped

2 garlic cloves, finely chopped

Directions:

1. Rinse the meat under running water and pat dry with a kitchen paper. Remove the bones and trim off the excess fat. Cut into bite-sized pieces and set aside.
2. Plug in your Instant Pot and add butter to the stainless steel insert. Press the Sauté button and stir with a wooden spatula until butter has completely melted.
3. Add meat, onions, and garlic. Sprinkle with some salt and cook for 5 minutes, stirring occasionally.
4. Add parsnips, carrot, and potatoes. Sprinkle with cayenne pepper and stir well.
5. Finally, add diced tomatoes and pour in the beef broth and 1 cup of water. Sprinkle with parsley, rosemary, and throw in the bay leaf. Stir well and securely lock the lid. Adjust the steam release handle and press the Manual button.
6. Set the timer for 25 minutes and cook on High pressure.
7. When done, perform a quick pressure release and open the pot.
8. Transfer to a serving dish and serve immediately. Enjoy!

Freestyle SmartPoints Per Serving: 4

(Calories 244 | Total Fats 8.2g | Net Carbs: 9.4g | Protein 29g | Fiber: 3.2g)

VEGETABLES AND VEGETARIAN DISHES

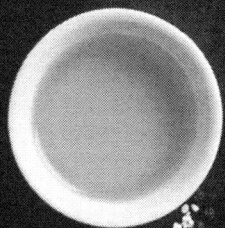

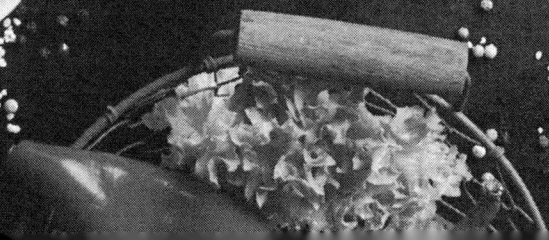

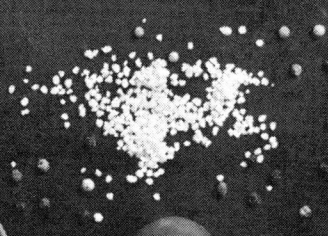

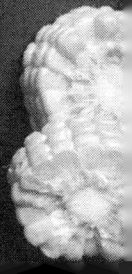

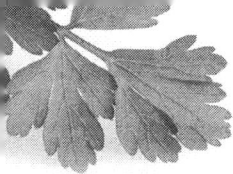

Farmer-Style Quiche

(Prep Time: 15 MIN | Cook Time: 45 MIN | Serves: 8)

Ingredients:

For cooking:

Nonstick spray

For quiche:

1 ready-made pie crust dough

⅓ cup onions (peeled, diced)

½ cup mushrooms (chopped)

1 cup organic spinach (chopped)

4 medium, free-range eggs

⅓ cup low-fat cottage cheese (grated)

⅓ cup low-fat Cheddar cheese (grated)

Sea salt and black pepper

¼ cup asiago cheese (grated)

Directions:

1. Preheat the main oven to 350 degrees F.
2. Roll out the pie crust and arrange in a 9" pie dish. Trim off any overhang and using a knife, make two small slits in the bottom of the pie crust; this will stop any air pockets from forming.
3. Cook in the preheated oven for 6 minutes and put to one side.
4. Add the onions, mushrooms, and spinach to a frying pan coated with nonstick spray and over moderate heat, cook for several minutes.
5. In the meantime, whisk the eggs in a bowl together with the cottage cheese. Add the grated Cheddar and season with a little salt and pepper.
6. Add the asiago cheese to the bottom of the pie crust.
7. Spoon on the onion-spinach mixture and top with the egg mixture.
8. Bake in the preheated oven for 40-45 minutes, or until sufficiently set.
9. Slice and serve.

Freestyle SmartPoints Per Serving: 5

(Calories 177 | Total Fats 10.9g | Net Carbs: 13.8g | Protein 6.2g | Fiber: 0g)

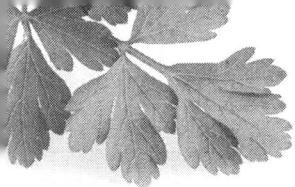

Homemade Ratatouille

(Prep Time: 15 MIN | Cook Time: 40 MIN | Serves: 6)

Ingredients:

For cooking:
2 tbsp olive oil

For vegetables:
½ pound eggplant (sliced)

½ pound zucchini (sliced)

½ pound Roma tomatoes (sliced)

2 garlic cloves (peeled, minced)

For seasoning:
Salt and black pepper

Pinch crushed red pepper

¼ cup red wine vinegar

2 tbsp fresh marjoram leaves (chopped)

Directions:

1. Preheat the main oven to 400 degrees F. Lightly grease a casserole dish with oil.
2. Arrange the vegetables in the dish.
3. In a bowl, combine the seasoning ingredients and sprinkle over the vegetables.
4. Bake in the preheated oven for 40-45 minutes, or until the veggies are fork-tender. Enjoy.

Freestyle SmartPoints Per Serving: 2

(Calories 68 | Total Fats 5g | Net Carbs: 4g | Protein 2g | Fiber: 2g)

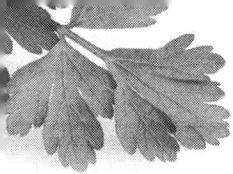

Old-Fashioned Green Bean Casserole

(Prep Time: 10 MIN | Cook Time: 25 MIN | Serves: 13)

Ingredients:

For cooking:

Nonstick cooking spray

For casserole:

3 (14½ ounce) cans French-
style green beans

1 (10½ ounce) can 98% fat-
free cream of mushroom
soup

½ cup skim milk

3 tbsp onion (peeled,
chopped)

¾ cup low-fat Cheddar
(shredded)

15 buttery, small circular
crackers

2 ounces French fried onions

2 tbsp light butter

Directions:

1. Preheat the main oven to 350 degrees F. Spritz a baking dish with nonstick spray.
2. Add the beans, soup, milk, onions, and cheese to the dish. Mix well to combine.
3. In a Ziplock bag, combine the crackers with the French fried onions and crush.
4. Transfer the crushed cracker mixture to a bowl.
5. In the microwave, melt the butter for 25 seconds.
6. Using a fork, stir the butter into the crushed cracker mixture, until incorporated.
7. Evenly spoon the butter mixture over the bean mixture in the baking dish.
8. Transfer the dish to the preheated oven and cook, uncovered, until the topping is golden, for 20-25 minutes. Serve.

Freestyle SmartPoints Per Serving: 3

(Calories 115 | Total Fats 6g | Net Carbs: 9g | Protein 4g | Fiber: 4g)

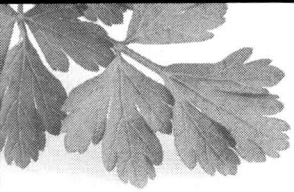

Pear and Prosciutto Stuffing with Hazelnuts

(Prep Time: 20 MIN | Cook Time: 1 HOUR 15 MIN | Serves: 12)

Ingredients:

For cooking:
Nonstick spray

Nonstick butter-
flavored cooking spray

2 tbsp light butter

For stuffing:
6 ounces prosciutto
(thinly sliced, cut into
bite-sized pieces)

8 cups stale multi-grain
baguette (cut into ½"
cubes)

3 small ripe, firm pears
(cored, chopped)

⅓ cup toasted
hazelnuts (chopped)

1 (14 ounce) can low-salt
chicken broth

¼ cup liquid egg
substitute

For vegetables:
1 cup celery (chopped)

2 cups yellow onion
(peeled, chopped)

2 cups fennel bulb
(diced)

¼ cup shallot (minced)

For seasoning:
2 tsp fresh sage
(minced)

1 tsp fresh rosemary
(minced)

2 tsp fresh thyme
(minced)

½ tsp salt

¼ tsp black pepper

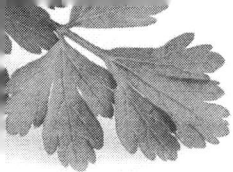

Directions:

1. Preheat the main oven to 350 degrees F. Spritz a 13x9" casserole dish with nonstick spray.
2. Spritz a frying pan with butter-flavored nonstick spray and over moderate heat. Cook the prosciutto, stirring until crisp, about 5 minutes. When sufficiently cooked, transfer to a plate lined with kitchen paper.
3. Using the same frying pan, melt the butter and add the vegetables, cook while stirring for 5-7 minutes.
4. Stir in the seasoning and cook for 60 seconds.
5. Transfer the mixture to a mixing bowl and stir in the cubes of bread, followed by the pears, hazelnuts, and crisp prosciutto.
6. Pour in the broth and add the egg substitute, toss well to combine evenly.
7. Transfer the mixture to the casserole dish and cover with aluminum foil.
8. Bake in the preheated oven for 40 minutes, before removing the aluminum foil.
9. Return to the oven and bake for another 25-30 minutes, or until the top is starting to crisp. Serve.

Freestyle SmartPoints Per Serving: 4

(Calories 156 | Total Fats 4g | Net Carbs: 20g | Protein 9g | Fiber: 6g)

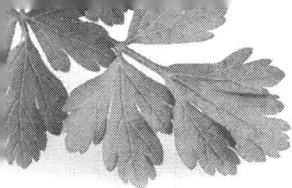

Potato and Cauliflower Curry

(Prep Time: 15 MIN | Cook Time: 30 MIN | Serves: 6)

Ingredients:

For spice paste:

1 inch piece ginger (peeled, grated)

½ tsp red pepper flakes

½ tsp red pepper flakes

2 garlic cloves (peeled, minced)

2 tbsp vegetable oil

2 tsp cumin

1 tbsp coriander

2 tsp turmeric

½ tsp salt

For curry:

1½ pounds potatoes (peeled, cubed)

1 head cauliflower florets (trimmed)

1¼ cups water

½ cup fresh cilantro (roughly chopped, to garnish)

Directions:

1. Combine spice paste ingredients in a small bowl.
2. Heat a pan over low heat, before adding the spice paste. Cook for 4-5 minutes, until the spices emit their fragrance. Add the potatoes and florets, bring to a moderate heat and stir well for a few minutes.
3. Pour in the water, mix to combine, cover and simmer until fork-tender; this will take between 20-25 minutes.
4. Serve, garnished with chopped cilantro.

Freestyle SmartPoints Per Serving: 4

(Calories 137 | Total Fats 5g | Net Carbs: 17.5g | Protein 3g | Fiber: 4g)

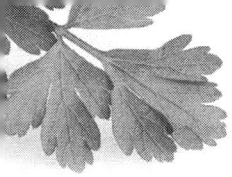

Spanish Potato and Onion Tortilla

(Prep Time: 10 MIN | Cook Time: 40 MIN | Serves: 6)

Ingredients:

For cooking:

2 tbsp olive oil

For the tortilla:

1½ pounds potatoes
(chopped into small cubes)
1 onion (peeled, thinly sliced)
8 medium eggs
Sea salt and black pepper

Directions:

1. Preheat the main oven to 400 degrees F.
2. Over moderate heat in an ovenproof pan, heat the oil. Add the potatoes, followed by the onion and cook for 15-20 minutes, until fork-tender, while frequently stirring.
3. In the meantime, whisk the eggs in a bowl and season.
4. Add whisked eggs to the pan, using a spatula, firmly press the mixture into an even layer. Cook for a few minutes before transferring to the oven for 5-7 minutes, until sufficiently cooked.

Freestyle SmartPoints Per Serving: 4

(Calories 231 | Total Fats 11g | Net Carbs: 19g | Protein 11g | Fiber: 3g)

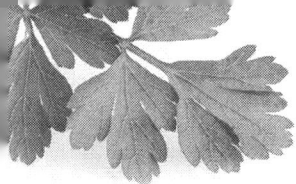

Strawberry and Almond Avocado Salad

(Prep Time: 10 MIN | Cook Time: N/A | Serves: 4)

Ingredients:

For salad:

5 cups kale (chopped)

½ cup strawberries (hulled, sliced)

½ ripe avocado (peeled, pitted, chopped)

¼ almonds (sliced)

For dressing:

2 tbsp virgin olive oil

Freshly squeezed juice from 1 medium lemon

1 tbsp runny honey

Salt and black pepper

Directions:

1. In a serving bowl, add all of the salad ingredients, toss to combine.

2. In a small jug, whisk the dressing ingredients together until combined.

3. Pour the dressing over the salad and toss to coat. Serve.

Freestyle SmartPoints Per Serving: 7

(Calories 214 | Total Fats 15g | Net Carbs: 12g | Protein 6g | Fiber: 6g)

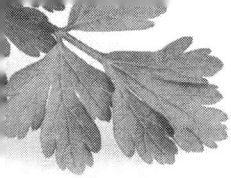

Egg, Tomato, and Cheese Supper Mug

(Prep Time: 1 MIN | Cook Time: 3 MIN | Serves: 1)

Ingredients:

For cooking:

Nonstick spray

For supper mug:

1 medium egg

Whites of 2 medium eggs

½ cup fresh tomatoes
(diced)

1 tbsp basil

1 tbsp Parmesan cheese
(freshly grated)

Kosher salt and black
pepper

Directions:

1. Spritz a large coffee mug with nonstick spray.
2. In a bowl whisk the eggs with the egg whites. Stir in the tomatoes along with the basil, grated cheese, kosher salt and black pepper.
3. Pour into the mug and microwave in 20-25 second intervals for 2-3 minutes until cooked through.

Freestyle Smart Points Per Serving: 1

(Calories 148 | Total Fats 7g | Net Carbs: 2g | Protein 17g | Fiber: 1g)

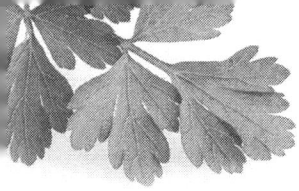

Greek Feta and Veggie Frittata

(Prep Time: 10 MIN | Cook Time: 35 MIN | Serves: 6)

Ingredients:

For cooking:

1 tbsp virgin olive oil

For frittata:

3 cups asparagus (chopped)

1½ cups mushrooms (sliced)

3 scallions (chopped)

1 clove garlic (peeled, minced)

Sea salt and black pepper

12 medium eggs

¾ cup reduced fat milk

1 cup reduced-fat Greek feta cheese

Directions:

1. Preheat the main oven to 400 degrees F.
2. In a skillet over moderately high heat, heat the olive oil.
3. Add the chopped asparagus along with the mushrooms and scallions. Cook until fork-tender, for between 5-7 minutes. Add the garlic and cook for 60 seconds, until fragrant. Season with sea salt and black pepper.
4. In a bowl, combine the eggs, and milk, whisking to incorporate.
5. Add the cooked vegetables and feta cheese to the bottom of pie plate.
6. Pour the egg mixture over the vegetables and cheese and stir to incorporate.
7. Bake in the oven for between 20-30 minutes until the eggs are sufficiently set and cooked through.

Freestyle Smart Points Per Serving: 3

(Calories 242 | Total Fats 15g | Net Carbs: 5g | Protein 20g | Fiber: 2g)

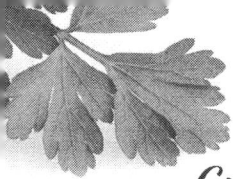

Grilled Portobello Mushroom Burgers with Swiss Cheese

(Prep Time: 15 MIN | Cook Time: 15 MIN | Serves: 4)

Ingredients:

For marinating:

2 tbsp balsamic vinegar

1 tbsp olive oil

1 tbsp Worcestershire sauce

1 tbsp Italian seasoning mix

1½ steak seasoning

For burgers:

4 Portobello mushrooms
(caps only)

1 red onion (peeled, sliced)

4 slices Jarlsberg cheese

4 low-calorie hamburger
buns (halved)

1 large tomato (sliced)

1 avocado (peeled, pitted,
sliced)

2 cups arugula

Directions:

1. Combine the marinating ingredients in a medium bowl. Add the mushroom caps to the marinating liquid and set to one side for an hour.
2. Preheat a grill for direct heat.
3. Remove the mushrooms from the marinating liquid and gently shake to remove any excess liquid. Place on the grill and cook for 4 minutes on each side. At the same time, add the onions to the grill and cook until softened.
4. For the final minute of grilling, lay a cheese slice on top of each mushroom and allow to melt a little.
5. Place one cheesy mushroom into each hamburger bun and top each with an equal amount of grilled onion, sliced tomato, avocado, and arugula.

Freestyle Smart Points Per Serving: 7

(Calories 300 | Total Fats 13g | Net Carbs: 27g | Protein 15g | Fiber: 9g)

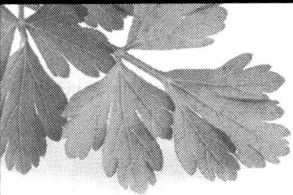

Healthy Eggplant and Spinach Italian Rollatini

(Prep Time: 25 MIN | Cook Time: 1 HOUR 25 MIN | Serves: 5)

Ingredients:

For rollatini:

2 medium Italian eggplants

Sea salt

Black pepper

1½ cups jarred marinara sauce

1 cup semi-skim mozzarella cheese (shredded)

For spinach filling:

1 large egg (beaten)

½ cup semi-skim ricotta cheese

½ cup Pecorino Romano cheese (grated)

8 ounces frozen spinach

1 clove garlic (peeled, minced)

¼ tsp kosher salt

⅛ tsp black pepper

Directions:

1. Cut both ends off each eggplant. Using a mandolin, cut the eggplants across their length into 10 (¼") thick slices.
2. Sprinkle the eggplant with salt as this will help to negate the eggplant's bitter taste. Set to one side for 10-15 minutes before patting dry using kitchen paper towel.
3. Preheat the main oven to 400 degrees F.
4. Season the eggplant with a pinch more salt and a dash of pepper. Arrange the eggplant on 2 baking sheets, lined with parchment paper. Tightly cover with aluminum foil and bake for 8-10 minutes, until the eggplant is pliable, tender but not thoroughly cooked.
5. Ladle ¼ cup of the marinara sauce into the bottom of a 13x9" casserole dish.
6. In a mixing bowl, combine all spinach filling ingredients.
7. Using kitchen paper towel pat the eggplant dry.
8. Evenly divide and spoon the spinach mixture over the eggplant and spread to cover.
9. Beginning at the shorter end, roll up the slices and arrange in the casserole dish, seam side facing down.
10. Spoon on the remaining marinara sauce along with the mozzarella and using aluminum foil, tightly cover.
11. Bake in the preheated oven until fork tender, for around 1 hour.
12. Remove and set aside to cool for 5 minutes.
13. Serve.

Freestyle Smart Points Per Serving: 5

(Calories 227 | Total Fats 10g | Net Carbs: 13g | Protein 17g | Fiber: 5g)

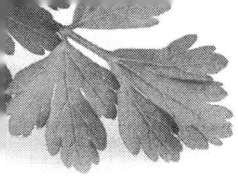

Herby Greek Salad with Quinoa

(Prep Time: 10 MIN | Cook Time: N/A | Serves: 4)

Ingredients:

For salad:

3 cups cooked quinoa

1 (14 ounce) can cannellini beans (drained, rinsed)

2 cups tomatoes (diced)

1 cup red onion (peeled, finely chopped)

2 cups cucumber (finely chopped)

4 radishes (chopped)

½ cup fresh parsley (roughly chopped)

¼ cup fresh mint (roughly chopped)

¼ cup fresh basil (roughly chopped)

½ cup pitted Kalamata olives (thinly sliced)

For dressing:

Juice and zest of 1 medium lemon

2 tbsp extra virgin olive oil

Sea salt and black pepper

Directions:

1. Add all salad ingredients to a large bowl and toss to combine.
2. Combine the dressing ingredients in a small bowl and drizzle over the salad. Toss again to evenly distribute the dressing and serve.

Freestyle Smart Points Per Serving: 7

(Calories 396 | Total Fats 12g | Net Carbs: 49g | Protein 16g | Fiber: 12g)

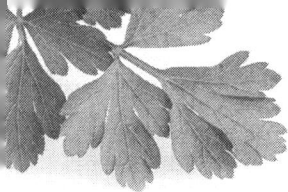

Moo Shu Stir-Fry

(Prep Time: 10 MIN | Cook Time: 15 MIN | Serves: 5)

Ingredients:

For cooking:
Nonstick spray
2 tsp sesame oil

For sauce:
½ cup hoisin sauce
2 tsp sesame oil
3 tsp garlic (peeled, minced)
2 tsp fresh ginger (peeled, minced)
2 tsp rice vinegar
1 tsp Asian hot sauce

For stir-fry:
4 medium eggs (beaten)
3 cups chopped cabbage slaw mix
1 (14 ounce) can Asian mixed vegetables (drained)
6 scallions (chopped)
4 tbsp water
3 tbsp fresh cilantro (minced)

Directions:

1. Whisk together all sauce ingredients in a small bowl and set to one side.
2. Spritz a skillet with nonstick spray and pour in the sesame oil, place over high heat.
3. Add the beaten egg to the skillet and cook until scrambled, set the cooked egg to one side.
4. Using the same skillet add the remaining stir-fry ingredients and cook for 4-5 minutes, until the vegetables are tender.
5. Pour in the set-aside sauce and toss well to coat the vegetables, cook for 2 minutes until hot through.
6. Return the set aside egg to the wok, stir until incorporated and serve hot.

Freestyle Smart Points Per Serving: 3

(Calories 208 | Total Fats 8g | Net Carbs: 19g | Protein 7g | Fiber: 5g)

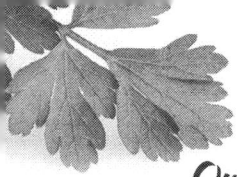

Orzo Dinner Salad with Feta Cheese and Greek Dressing

(Prep Time: 1 HOUR 10 MIN | Cook Time: 10 MIN | Serves: 3)

Ingredients:

For salad:

4 ounces dry whole wheat orzo

⅓ cup grape tomatoes (diced)

⅓ cup cucumbers (diced)

6 Kalamata olives (pitted, sliced)

2 ounces Feta cheese (crumbled)

For dressing:

1 tbsp Greek olive oil

4 tsp white wine vinegar

¼ tsp garlic powder

¼ tsp onion powder

¼ tsp dried basil

¼ tsp dried oregano

¼ tsp sea salt

¼ tsp freshly ground black pepper

¼ tsp yellow mustard

Directions:

1. Cook the orzo according to package instructions and thoroughly drain. Set to one side to cool and then store in a re-sealable container in the fridge for a minimum of 60 minutes.

2. As soon as the orzo is cooled, transfer to a mixing bowl along with all remaining salad ingredients, toss together until combined.

3. In a second bowl, combine the dressing ingredients and stir well to incorporate.

4. Pour the dressing over the orzo salad and toss until evenly coated.

Freestyle Smart Points Per Serving: 8

(Calories 250 | Total Fats 10g | Net Carbs: 26g | Protein 8g | Fiber: 4g)

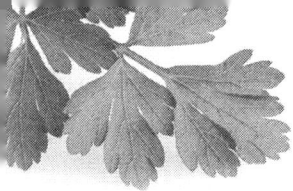

Oven-Roasted Vegetable Fajitas

(Prep Time: 10 MIN | Cook Time: 20 MIN | Serves: 4)

Ingredients:

For vegetables:

2 medium zucchini (halved lengthwise, sliced)

2 medium carrots (peeled, sliced)

1 red bell pepper (sliced into strips)

1 green bell pepper (sliced into strips)

1 red onion (peeled, sliced)

1 cup sweet corn

1 tbsp freshly squeezed lime juice

1 tbsp olive oil

Seasoning:

1 tsp smoked paprika

1 tsp ground coriander

1 tsp kosher salt

1 tsp powdered garlic

1 tsp hot chili powder

1 tsp ground cumin

½ tsp black pepper

For serving:

¼ cup fresh cilantro (roughly chopped)

8 (8") corn tortillas (warmed)

½ cup low-fat Cheddar cheese (shredded)

½ cup tomato salsa

Directions:

1. Preheat the main oven to 500 degrees F. Line a baking sheet with aluminum foil.
2. Add all of the vegetable ingredients to a large bowl and toss well to combine.
3. Sprinkle the vegetable mixture with the seasoning and toss again until the vegetable mixture is evenly coated.
4. Transfer the mixture to the baking sheet and spread out into an even layer.
5. Place in the oven and bake for just under 20 minutes. Scatter with the fresh cilantro.
6. Divide the fajita mixture between the warmed tortillas and serve with the shredded cheese and tomato salsa.

Freestyle Smart Points Per Serving: 6

(Calories 281 | Total Fats 7g | Net Carbs: 37g | Protein 12g | Fiber: 9g)

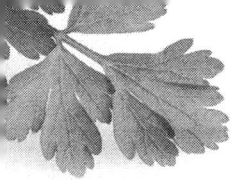

Sweet Potato and Chickpea Casserole

(Prep Time: 15 MIN | Cook Time: 7 HOUR 15 MIN | Serves: 6)

Ingredients:

For casserole:

1 medium yellow onion
(peeled, chopped)
2 (15-ounce) cans garbanzo
beans (drained)
1 pound sweet potatoes
(peeled, chopped)
1 tbsp garlic (peeled,
minced)
4 cups fat-free vegetable
broth

Seasoning:

½ tsp kosher salt
¼ tsp coarse black pepper
1tsp ground ginger
1½ tsp ground cumin
1 tsp ground coriander
¼ tsp ground cinnamon

For serving:

4 cups fresh baby spinach

Directions:

1. In a microwave-safe bowl, microwave the onions for 2-3 minutes.
2. Transfer the onions to a slow cooker along with the remaining casserole ingredients. Stir well and add the seasoning stir again and cover. Cook for 6-7 hours on low heat.
3. Stir in the spinach leaves and cook for a final 10 minutes before serving.

Freestyle Smart Points Per Serving: 3

(Calories 165 | Total Fats 2g | Net Carbs: 26g | Protein 6.5g | Fiber: 6g)

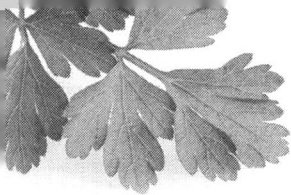

Tex Mex Black Bean Stuffed Squash

(Prep Time: 15 MIN | Cook Time: 45 MIN | Serves: 4)

Ingredients:

For squash:

4 summer squash (halved)

2 cups canned black beans (drained, rinsed)

1 clove garlic (peeled, minced)

½ cup red bell pepper (seeded, diced)

1 cup yellow onion (peeled, minced)

½ cup low-fat Cheddar cheese (shredded)

For sauce:

½ tsp cumin

Salt and black pepper

1 cup jarred enchilada sauce

Directions:

1. Preheat the main oven to 400 degrees F.
2. Scoop out the flesh from the halves of squash. Chop the squash flesh and transfer to a skillet over moderate heat.
3. Add the black beans, garlic, bell pepper, and onion to the skillet and sauté for several minutes.
4. Combine the sauce ingredients in a small bowl, stir well and then pour into the skillet. Stir again to combine and then take the skillet off the heat.
5. Spoon the mixture into the squash halves and scatter each with an equal amount of shredded cheese.
6. Arrange the stuffed squashes on a baking tray and loosely tent with aluminum foil. Place in the oven and bake for 25 minutes, discard the foil and cook for a final 10 minutes. Allow to cool for a few minutes before serving.

Freestyle Smart Points Per Serving: 3

(Calories 220 | Total Fats 2g | Net Carbs: 23g | Protein 15g | Fiber: 13g)

INSTANT POT
VEGETARIAN DISHES

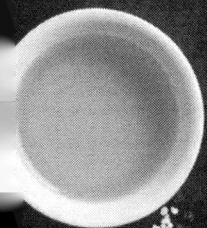

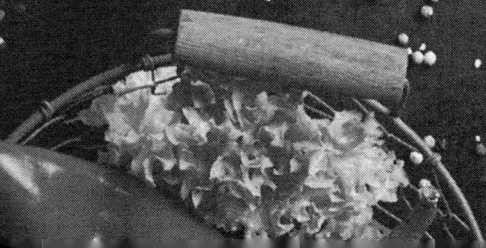

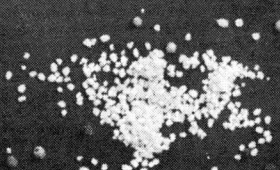

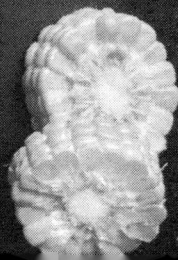

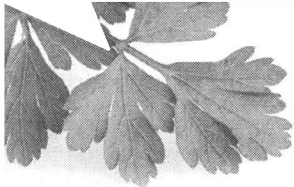

Quinoa with Eggplant and Lime

(Prep Time: 10 MIN | Cook Time: 6 MIN | Serves: 4)

Ingredients:

For cooking:

2 tsp olive oil

For salad:

1 cup white quinoa

1 medium-sized eggplant, cut into cubes

1 cup fennel, chopped

1 small carrot, sliced

1 small onion, chopped

1 tbsp fresh parsley, finely chopped

2 tsp fresh lime juice

Seasoning:

1 tsp dried rosemary, ground

½ tsp dried marjoram, ground

Salt

Black pepper

Directions:

1. Plug in the instant pot and place quinoa in the stainless steel insert. Pour in 1 ¼ cup of water and sprinkle with some salt. Securely lock the lid and adjust the steam release handle. Press the Manual button and set the timer for 1 minute. Cook on High pressure.

2. When done, perform a quick pressure release and open the pot. Transfer to a bowl and cover with a lid.

3. Now, grease the stainless steel insert with olive oil. Press the Sauté button and add eggplant, carrot, fennel, and onion. Sprinkle with salt, rosemary, marjoram, and pepper. Stir-fry for 5 minutes, or until softened.

4. Stir in the quinoa, lime juice, and parsley. Turn off the pot and transfer all to a serving bowl.

5. Let it chill for 15 minutes before serving.

Freestyle SmartPoints Per Serving: 6

(Calories 238 | Total Fats 5.1g | Net Carbs: 31g | Protein 7.7g | Fiber: 8.4g)

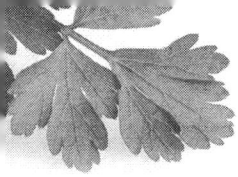

Crust-less Vegetable Flan

(Prep Time: 15 MIN | Cook Time: 6 MIN | Serves: 4)

Ingredients:

For cooking:
2 tsp olive oil

For flan:
1 medium-sized zucchini, chopped
2 small onions, chopped
2 spring onions, chopped
3 red bell peppers, chopped
1 cup cauliflower, chopped
1 cup cottage cheese
¼ cup skim milk
¼ cup fresh parsley, finely chopped
2 large eggs, beaten

Seasoning:
Salt
Black pepper

Directions:

1. In a medium-sized mixing bowl, combine eggs, milk, cheese, and parsley. Mix until well blended. Add all remaining vegetables and sprinkle with some salt and pepper. Stir until all well combined.
2. Plug in the instant pot and grease the stainless steel insert with olive oil. Pour in the previously prepared mixture and securely lock the lid. Adjust the steam release handle by moving the valve to the Sealing position. Press the Manual button and set the timer for 6 minutes. Cook on High pressure.
3. When you hear the cooker's end signal, perform a quick pressure release and open the pot.
4. Transfer to a serving dish and garnish with some fresh cilantro. Enjoy!

Freestyle SmartPoints Per Serving: 3

(Calories 173 | Total Fats 6.3g | Net Carbs: 13.4g | Protein 14g | Fiber: 3.4g)

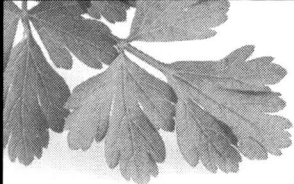

Ratatouille

(Prep Time: 15 MIN | Cook Time: 18 MIN | Serves: 3)

Ingredients:

For cooking:

2 tsp olive oil

For ratatouille:

2 cups tomatoes, diced

½ eggplant, chopped

1 small onion, chopped

2 bell peppers, chopped

3 garlic cloves, chopped

¼ zucchini, chopped

2 tbsp red wine vinegar

Seasoning:

1 tsp dried marjoram, ground

1 bay leaf

Salt

Pepper

Directions:

1. Preheat the oven to 400 degrees. Line a large baking sheet with some parchment paper and set aside.
2. Dice the tomatoes and spread over the baking sheet in one thin layer. Place in the oven and roast for 10 minutes. When done, remove to a wire rack and set aside.
3. Plug in your Instant Pot and grease the stainless steel insert with olive oil. Add eggplant, onions, bell peppers, and zucchini. Cook for 5 minutes, stirring occasionally.
4. Now, sprinkle with red wine vinegar, marjoram, salt, and pepper. Stir in the roasted tomatoes and pour in ½ cup of water. Securely lock the lid and adjust the steam release handle. Press the Manual button and set the timer for 3 minutes. Cook on High pressure.
5. When you hear the cooker's end signal, perform a quick pressure release and open the pot.
6. Sprinkle with some fresh parsley before serving.

Freestyle SmartPoints Per Serving: 1

(Calories 111 | Total Fats 3.8g | Net Carbs: 13.1g | Protein 3.3g | Fiber: 5.9g)

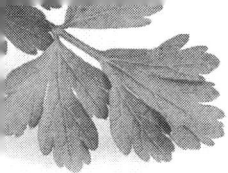

Marinated Broccoli

(Prep Time: 15 MIN | Cook Time: 18 MIN | Serves: 2)

Ingredients:

For cooking:

3 cups vegetable broth, low-sodium

For broccoli:

1 lb broccoli, cut into bite-sized pieces
1 tsp lemon juice
1 tsp salt
½ tsp black pepper

For marinade:

2 tsp olive oil
1 tbsp dry sherry
½ tsp Worcestershire sauce
½ tsp Dijon mustard
½ tsp dried thyme, ground

Directions:

1. Place the broccoli in a large colander. Rinse well under cold running water. Drain well and transfer to a cutting board. Cut into bite-sized pieces and place in a large bowl. Sprinkle with some salt, pepper, and lemon juice. Set aside.

2. In a small bowl, combine all marinade ingredients. Mix until well combined and drizzle over the broccoli. Toss well and let it stand for 20-30 minutes. Stir occasionally.

3. Plug in the Instant Pot and pour the vegetable broth into the stainless steel insert. Add marinated broccoli with all the remaining liquid. Securely lock the lid and adjust the steam release handle.

4. Press the Manual button and cook for 4 minutes on High pressure.

5. When done, perform a quick pressure release and open the pot. Transfer all to a serving plate and optionally, top with some low-fat cream cheese. Enjoy!

Freestyle SmartPoints Per Serving: 3

(Calories 184 | Total Fats 7.6g | Net Carbs: 11.1g | Protein 13.8g | Fiber: 6.2g)

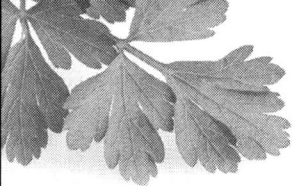

Wild Rice Mushroom Stir-Fry

(Prep Time: 5 MIN | Cook Time: 12 MIN | Serves: 3)

Ingredients:

For cooking:

2 cups vegetable broth

1 tsp butter

For stir-fry:

8 oz button mushrooms, sliced

1 cup wild rice

½ cup green peas

½ cup celery, chopped

1 small onion, chopped

2 garlic cloves, minced

Seasoning:

½ tsp dried thyme, ground

¼ tsp dried oregano, ground

½ tsp cayenne pepper

Salt

Pepper

Directions:

1. Plug in the instant pot and place the butter in the stainless steel insert. Melt over the Sauté mode, stirring gently.

2. Add onions, garlic, and mushrooms. Cook for 5 minutes, or until the mushrooms soften.

3. Now, add wild rice, celery, and green peas. Sprinkle with thyme, oregano, salt, and pepper. Pour in the broth and give it a good stir. Securely lock the lid and adjust the steam release handle.

4. Press the Manual button and set the timer for 3 minutes. Cook on High pressure.

5. When you hear the cooker's end signal, perform a quick pressure release and open the pot. Press the Sauté button and continue to cook for 3-4 minutes more.

6. Transfer all to a serving plate and garnish with some lemon slices. Enjoy!

Freestyle SmartPoints Per Serving: 6

(Calories 278 | Total Fats 3.1g | Net Carbs: 45.8g | Protein 15.3g | Fiber: 6.1g)

SNACKS

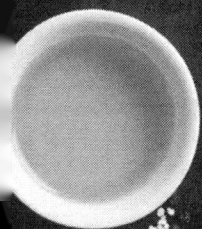
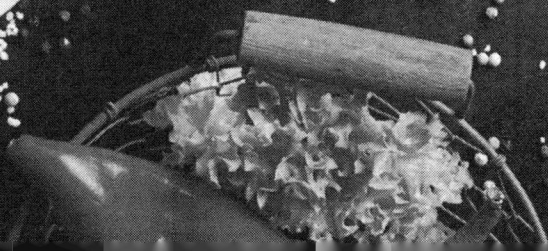
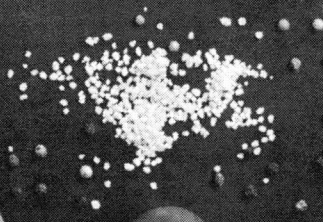
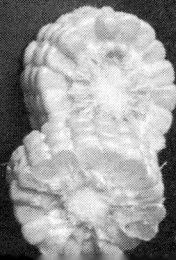

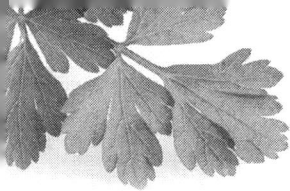

Asian Veggie Egg Rolls

(Prep Time: 25 MIN | Cook Time: 25 MIN | Serves: 12)

Ingredients:

For cooking:
Nonstick spray
1 tsp olive oil

For vegetables:
1 cup scallions (chopped)
1 cup carrot (peeled, grated)
2½ cups cabbage (shredded)
1 cup snow peas (finely chopped)
2½ cups broccoli slaw (no dressing)

For egg rolls:
2 cloves garlic (peeled, minced)
2 tsp jarred ginger (chopped)
Pinch black pepper
2 tbsp rice vinegar
1½ tbsp soy sauce
12 egg roll wrappers

Directions:

1. Preheat the main oven to 425 degrees F and spritz a baking sheet with nonstick spray, set to one side.
2. Add all of the vegetables to a large bowl and toss to combine.
3. Heat the oil in a skillet over moderately high heat and sauté the garlic and ginger for 40 seconds, before adding the vegetables, black pepper, rice vinegar, and soy sauce. Cook for several minutes, until softened but still a little crisp. Transfer to a bowl and chill for 15 minutes.
4. Taking one wrapper at a time, place a wrapper on a plate with the pointed side towards you.
5. Place a ⅓ of a cup of filling onto the center of the wrapper. Fold the bottom corner over the filling and then the left and right corners, then roll up to form an egg roll.
6. Repeat with the remaining wrappers and filling and arrange on the baking sheet.
7. Place in the oven and bake for 20 minutes, flipping the egg rolls over halfway through cooking. Serve hot.

Freestyle SmartPoints Per Serving: 3

(Calories 115 | Total Fats 3g | Net Carbs: 15g | Protein 6g | Fiber: 2g)

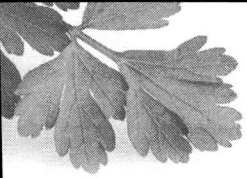

Baba Ganoush Eggplant Dip

(Prep Time: 10 MIN | Cook Time: 25 MIN | Serves: 6)

Ingredients:

For cooking:

Nonstick spray

For dip:

2 large eggplants (pierced all over with a fork)

1 tbsp low-fat mayo

3 cloves garlic (peeled, minced)

¼ cup fat-free plain Greek yogurt

1 tbsp tahini

Juice of 1 medium lemon

Sea salt and black pepper

Directions:

1. Preheat the main oven to 450 degrees F, cover a baking sheet with parchment and spritz with nonstick spray.
2. Place the whole eggplants on the baking sheet and roast for just over 20 minutes.
3. Slice the cooked eggplant in half and transfer to a colander, set aside for 5-6 minutes to allow any excess liquid to drain away.
4. Scoop the flesh from each eggplant half into a blender and discard the skins.
5. On pulse setting, mash the eggplant until chunky and thick.
6. Add all of the remaining dip ingredients to the blender and blitz until just combined.
7. Serve with your favorite Zero Point veggies.

Freestyle SmartPoints Per Serving: 1

(Calories 65 | Total Fats 2g | Net Carbs: 5g | Protein 3g | Fiber: 5g)

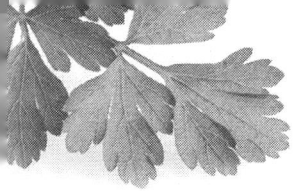

Blue Cheese Stuffed Celery Sticks

(Prep Time: 10 MIN | Cook Time: N/A | Serves: 4)

Ingredients:

For sauce:

⅓ cup hot sauce

½ tsp powdered garlic

2 tbsp low-fat cream cheese
(at room temperature)

For sticks:

4 celery stalks (sliced into 3
inch pieces)

2 cups cooked, shredded
chicken

2 tbsp low-fat ranch dressing

3 tbsp blue cheese (crumbled)

Directions:

1. Add all of the sauce ingredients to a bowl and stir until combined.
2. Add the chicken to the sauce and mix well.
3. Spoon the chicken mixture into the celery sticks and arrange on a serving plate.
4. Drizzle the ranch dressing over the sticks and sprinkle with the crumbled blue cheese. Enjoy!

Freestyle SmartPoints Per Serving: 2

(Calories 120 | Total Fats 5.5g | Net Carbs: 2.5g | Protein 13g | Fiber: 0.5g)

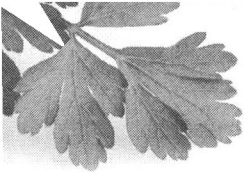

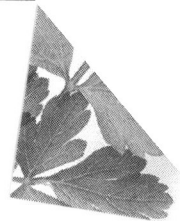

Butterscotch Pillows

(Prep Time: 10 MIN | Cook Time: 15 MIN | Serves: 64)

Ingredients:

For wet ingredients:

1 medium egg

½ cup low-calorie butter

1 cup brown sugar

1 tbsp canola oil

1 tsp vanilla essence

For dry ingredients:

1½ cups + 1 tbsp all-purpose flour

½ tsp kosher salt

½ tsp baking powder

¼ tsp bicarb of soda

1 cup crisp rice cereal

½ cup + 2 tbsp confectioner's sugar

Directions:

1. Preheat the main oven to 350 degrees F and cover a cookie sheet with parchment, set to one side.
2. Beat together all of the wet ingredients in a large bowl.
3. In a second bowl, combine all of the dry ingredients (excluding the cereal and sugar).
4. Add the dry ingredients to the wet, stirring until combined, then fold in the cereal.
5. Freeze the batter for half an hour.
6. Add the confectioner's sugar to a small bowl.
7. Take 1 tsp of the mixture at a time and roll into balls, then roll each ball in confectioner's sugar to coat, place on the cookie sheet.
8. Place in the oven and bake for just over 10 minutes, rotating the cookie sheet halfway through cooking.
9. Allow to cool completely before serving.

Freestyle SmartPoints Per Serving: 1

(Calories 40 | Total Fats 1g | Net Carbs: 7g | Protein 0g | Fiber: 0g)

Caesar Style Green Beans

(Prep Time: 10 MIN | Cook Time: 10 MIN | Serves: 4)

Ingredients:

For cooking:
Nonstick spray

For beans:
2 cups water
1 pound green beans
(trimmed)
1½ tbsp low-calorie Caesar
dressing
1 tbsp Parmesan cheese
(shredded)

For crumb topping:
1 slice wholegrain toast
1 tsp low-calorie butter
1 tsp powdered garlic

Directions:

1. Bring the water to a boil in a saucepan and add the green beans. Turn the heat down to a simmer, cover, and cook for several minutes, until tender, and drain.

2. In the meantime, spread the toast with the butter and sprinkle with powdered garlic. Pop in the microwave for 10 minutes and then transfer to a food processor, blitz until crumbed.

3. Transfer the green beans to a serving plate, sprinkle with the breadcrumbs, drizzle over the dressing and scatter with Parmesan.

4. Serve straight away.

Freestyle SmartPoints Per Serving: 2

(Calories 80 | Total Fats 3g | Net Carbs: 9g | Protein 4g | Fiber: 4g)

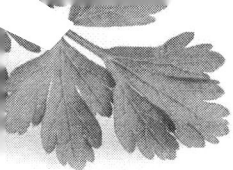

Mexican Street Style Corn

(Prep Time: 10 MIN | Cook Time: 10 MIN | Serves: 4)

Ingredients:

For cooking:
Nonstick spray

For corn:
4 ears fresh corn
Sea salt and black pepper
Wedge fresh lime
2 tbsp cotija cheese
(shredded)
½ tsp chili powder

For coating:
2 tbsp low-fat mayo
2 tbsp fat-free plain Greek
yogurt
Few dashes hot sauce

Directions:

1. Preheat your oven's broiler and cover a baking sheet with kitchen foil.
2. Spritz the corn ears with nonstick spray and place under the broiler. Broil for 10-12 minutes, flipping over halfway through cooking and then season with sea salt and black pepper.
3. In the meantime, combine all of the coating ingredients in a small bowl.
4. Spread 1 tbsp of coating mix onto each cooked ear of corn, squeeze over a little lime juice and sprinkle with chili powder.
5. Serve straight away.

Freestyle SmartPoints Per Serving: 4

(Calories 110 | Total Fats 4g | Net Carbs: 15g | Protein 4g | Fiber: 3g)

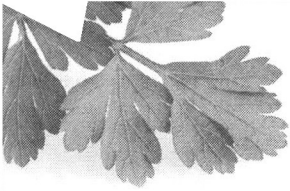

Moo Shu Lettuce Wraps

(Prep Time: 10 MIN | Cook Time: 15 MIN | Serves: 14)

Ingredients:

For cooking:
Nonstick spray

For wraps:
1 pound extra-lean ground turkey

14 Boston lettuce leaves

For vegetable mix:
½ cup + 2 tbsp hoisin sauce

1 tbsp jarred ginger

½ cup apple juice (unsweetened)

5 cups cabbage (shredded)

1½ cups carrot (peeled, shredded)

Directions:

1. Spritz a skillet with nonstick spray and place over moderately high heat.
2. Add the turkey and sauté until cooked through, using a wooden spoon to break up the turkey as it cooks.
3. Add all of the vegetable mix ingredients and stir well to combine, cook for 5 minutes, until the cabbage is softened but tender.
4. Spoon a ⅓ of a cup of turkey mixture into each lettuce leaf and serve straight away.

Freestyle SmartPoints Per Serving: 1

(Calories 75 | Total Fats 1g | Net Carbs: 7g | Protein 9g | Fiber: 1g)

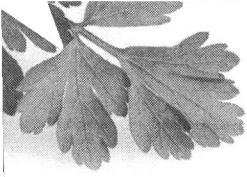

Rainbow Potato Salad

(Prep Time: 10 MIN | Cook Time: 15 MIN | Serves: 6)

Ingredients:

For potatoes:

1 pound yellow potatoes (cubed)

½ pound purple potatoes (cubed)

½ pound red potatoes (cubed)

For dressing:

1 celery stalk (finely chopped)

½ cup scallions (finely chopped)

½ cup fresh dill (roughly chopped)

Sea salt and black pepper

½ cup low-calorie ranch dressing

Directions:

1. Add the potatoes to a saucepan and completely cover with water. Bring to the boil, then cover and cook for 10-12 minutes at a simmer, until soft.
2. Drain the potatoes and set aside to cool.
3. In a serving bowl, add all of the dressing ingredients and stir to combine. Add the cooled potatoes and use a rubber spatula to mix until combined.
4. Chill until ready to serve.

Freestyle SmartPoints Per Serving: 4

(Calories 130 | Total Fats 1g | Net Carbs: 23g | Protein 4g | Fiber: 4g)

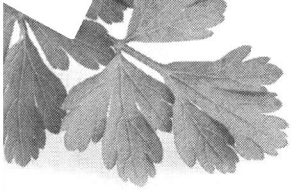

Spicy Ranch Onion Rings

(Prep Time: 10 MIN | Cook Time: 25 MIN | Serves: 10)

Ingredients:

For cooking:
Nonstick spray

For onion rings:
¼ cup flour

2 yellow onions (sliced into rings)

½ cup Panko breadcrumbs

For dip:
2 tbsp low-fat cream cheese (at room temperature)

2 tbsp low-calorie ranch dressing

2 tbsp hot sauce

Directions:

1. Preheat the main oven to 400 degrees F. Cover a baking sheet with kitchen foil.
2. Tip the flour into a large Ziplock bag and add the onion rings, shake to coat the onion in the flour.
3. Combine all of the dip ingredients in one shallow bowl and the breadcrumbs in a second one.
4. Dip each of the flour-coated onion rings first in the ranch mixture and then in the breadcrumbs.
5. Arrange the coated onions on the baking sheet and spritz generously with nonstick spray.
6. Bake in the oven for just over 20 minutes until golden. Enjoy warm.

Freestyle SmartPoints Per Serving: 1

(Calories 45 | Total Fats 1.5g | Net Carbs: 5g | Protein 1g | Fiber: 0g)

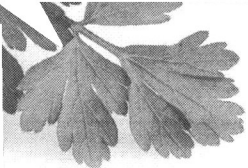

Chewy Marshmallow Cereal Squares

(Prep Time: 1 HOUR 10 MIN | Cook Time: 10 MIN | Serves: 16)

Ingredients:

For cooking:

Nonstick spray

For cereal squares:

2 tbsp margarine

10 ounces mini mallows

6 cups crispy rice cereal

Directions:

1. Spritz a rectangular glass baking dish with nonstick spray and set to one side.
2. In a saucepan over low heat, melt the margarine.
3. Add the mini mallows to the saucepan and cook gently, while stirring, until the mallows melt.
4. Take the saucepan off the heat and add the rice cereal. Stir well until the cereal is completely coated in the mallow mixture.
5. Transfer the mixture to the baking dish and press down, into all of the corners.
6. Chill for an hour before slicing into 16 equally-sized squares and serving.

Freestyle Smart Points Per Serving: 3

(Calories 85 | Total Fats 1g | Net Carbs: 19g | Protein 1g | Fiber: 0g)

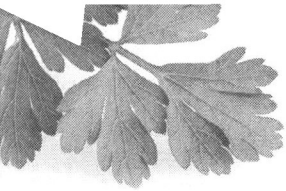

Cool Ranch Dip

(Prep Time: 5 MIN | Cook Time: N/A | Serves: 2)

Ingredients:

For ranch dip:

2 tbsp low-fat mayo

2 tbsp fat-free Greek yogurt

2 tbsp scallions (finely chopped)

Sea salt and black pepper

Directions:

1. In a small bowl, add all of the ingredients and stir to combine. Keep chilled until ready to serve and enjoy with your favorite ZeroPoint veggies.

Freestyle Smart Points Per Serving: 1

(Calories 41 | Total Fats 3.5g | Net Carbs: 1.5g | Protein 1g | Fiber: 0.2g)

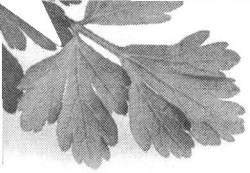

Cream Cheese Stuffed Bagel Balls

(Prep Time: 15 MIN | Cook Time: 25 MIN | Serves: 4)

Ingredients:

For cooking:
Nonstick spray

For dough balls:
2 tsp baking powder

¾ tsp kosher salt

1 cup all-purpose flour (unbleached)

1 cup non-fat plain Greek yogurt

4 ounces low-fat cream cheese (chopped into 8 cubes)

White of 1 medium egg (beaten)

Directions:

1. Preheat the main oven to 375 degrees F. Line a baking sheet with parchment and spritz with nonstick spray, set to one side.
2. Combine the baking powder, kosher salt, and flour in large bowl. Mix in the yogurt until well combined; the mixture will still be crumbly.
3. Lightly flour a worktop and knead the dough until tacky but not sticky (approximately 14 turns).
4. Split the dough into 8 equal portions and roll each portion into a ball. Flatten each ball and place a cube of cream cheese in the center. Fold the dough around the cheese and arrange on the baking sheet.
5. Brush the balls with beaten egg white.
6. Place in the oven and bake for just under half an hour.
7. Allow to cool before serving.

Freestyle Smart Points Per Serving: 5

(Calories 175 | Total Fats 3g | Net Carbs: 24g | Protein 10.5g | Fiber: 1g)

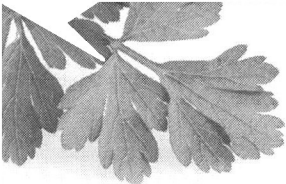

Feta, Olive, and Watermelon Wedges

(Prep Time: 10 MIN | Cook Time: N/A | Serves: 4)

Ingredients:

For watermelon:

8 (1" thick) wedges seedless
watermelon

1 ounce feta cheese
(crumbled)

5 pitted Kalamata olives (thinly
sliced)

1 tsp fresh mint (chopped)

½ tbsp balsamic glaze

Directions:

1. Arrange the watermelon wedges in a circle (like a pizza) on a serving plate.
2. Scatter with the crumbled feta cheese, sliced olives, and chopped mint.
3. Drizzle with balsamic glaze and enjoy.

Freestyle Smart Points Per Serving: 1

(Calories 90 | Total Fats 3g | Net Carbs: 13g | Protein 2g | Fiber: 1g)

Jalapeno Poppers

(Prep Time: 15 MIN | Cook Time: 30 MIN | Serves: 4)

Ingredients:

For cooking:
Nonstick spray

For filling:
2 ounces low-fat cream cheese (at room temperature)
½ cup low-fat Cheddar cheese (grated)
1 tbsp low-fat mayo

For jalapenos:
8 jalapeno peppers (sliced lengthwise, seeded)
¾ cup panko breadcrumbs.
¼ cup fat-free egg substitute

Directions:

1. Preheat the main oven to 350 degrees F Spritz a baking sheet with nonstick spray and set to one side.
2. Add the filling ingredients to a bowl and stir well to combine.
3. Spoon the filling mixture equally into the jalapeno halves.
4. Add the breadcrumbs and egg substitute to two shallow dishes.
5. Dip each stuffed jalapeno, first in the egg, and then in the breadcrumbs to coat.
6. Arrange on the baking sheet and place in the oven. Bake for half an hour until bubbling and golden. Allow to cool a little before serving.

Freestyle Smart Points Per Serving: 2

(Calories 160 | Total Fats 6g | Net Carbs: 16g | Protein 9g | Fiber: 2g)

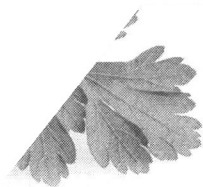

Parmesan Garlic Knots

(Prep Time: 20 MIN | Cook Time: 25 MIN | Serves: 8)

Ingredients:

For cooking:

Olive oil nonstick spray

For knots:

2 tsp baking powder

¾ tsp kosher salt

1 cup all-purpose flour (unbleached)

1 cup non-fat plain Greek yogurt

For garlic butter:

2 tsp salted butter

3 garlic cloves (peeled, finely chopped)

1 tbsp Parmesan cheese (grated)

1 tbsp fresh parsley (finely chopped)

Directions:

1. Preheat the main oven to 375 degrees F. Line a baking sheet with parchment and spritz with nonstick spray, set to one side.

2. Combine the baking powder, kosher salt, and flour in a large bowl. Mix in the yogurt until well combined; the mixture will still be crumbly.

3. Lightly flour a worktop and knead the dough until tacky but not sticky (approximately 14 turns).

4. Split the dough into 8 equally-sized portions. Roll each portion into a 9" log and tie each log into a loose knot. Arrange the knots on the baking sheet.

5. Spritz the knots with olive oil nonstick spray. Place in the oven and bake for just under 20 minutes, allow to cool for a few minutes.

6. Melt the butter in a skillet over moderate heat, add the garlic and sauté for 2 minutes until golden. Add the cooked knots to the skillet and toss to coat in the garlic butter. Transfer to a serving plate.

7. Sprinkle the Parmesan cheese and fresh parsley over the garlic knots and serve hot.

Freestyle Smart Points Per Serving: 2

(Calories 90 | Total Fats 1.5g | Net Carbs: 13.5g | Protein 5g | Fiber: 0.5g)

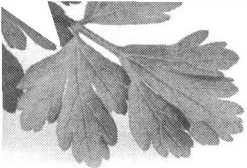

Pepperoni Pizza Zucchini Bites

(Prep Time: 10 MIN | Cook Time: 5 MIN | Serves: 2)

Ingredients:

For cooking:
Nonstick spray

For zucchini bites:
1 small zucchini (sliced
diagonally into ¼" pieces)
⅛ tsp garlic salt
¼ cup jarred marinara sauce
¼ cup semi-skim mozzarella
cheese (shredded)
¾ ounce turkey pepperoni
(chopped)

Directions:

1. Preheat the oven's broiler. Arrange a wire rack on an aluminum foil-lined baking sheet.
2. Spritz the zucchini slices with nonstick spray on both sides and arrange on the baking sheet in a single layer.
3. Sprinkle the zucchini with the garlic salt and place under the broiler for 4 minutes.
4. Remove from the oven and spoon 1 tsp of marinara sauce onto each zucchini slice and top with 1 tsp shredded cheese. Sprinkle with the chopped turkey pepperoni.
5. Place back under the broiler for 1-2 minutes more until the cheese has melted a little.
6. Serve hot.

Freestyle Smart Points Per Serving: 2

(Calories 72 | Total Fats 3g | Net Carbs: 5g | Protein 5.5g | Fiber: 1.5g)

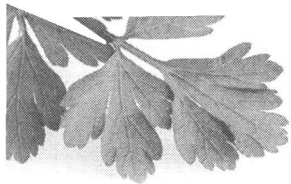

Prosciutto Wrapped Figs

(Prep Time: 10 MIN | Cook Time: N/A | Serves: 2)

Ingredients:

For wrapped figs:

1 ounce prosciutto (sliced into 8 pieces)

4 fresh figs (halved)

Black pepper

Directions:

1. Wrap 1 slice of prosciutto around each fig half and arrange on a plate. Sprinkle with black pepper and serve.

Freestyle Smart Points Per Serving: 1

(Calories 110 | Total Fats 1g | Net Carbs: 20g | Protein 5g | Fiber: 4g)

INSTANT POT SNACKS

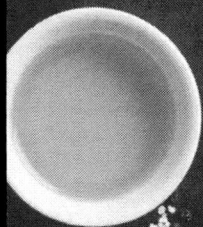

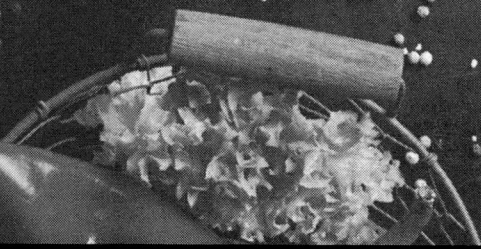

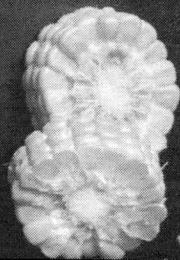

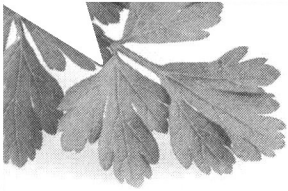

Fried Zucchini Toast

(Prep Time: 10 MIN | Cook Time: 6-8 MIN | Serves: 2)

Ingredients:

For cooking:

1 tbsp olive oil

For toast:

4 slices whole grain bread

½ zucchini, sliced

Seasoning:

¼ tsp dried marjoram

¼ tsp dried rosemary

½ tsp salt

¼ tsp black pepper

Directions:

12. Thinly slice zucchini and sprinkle with salt, rosemary, and marjoram. Set aside.
13. Plug in the Instant Pot and press the Sauté button. Grease the inner pot with olive oil and heat up.
14. Add zucchini slices and cook for 3-4 minutes on each side. Remove from the pot and divide between bread slices.
15. Sprinkle with some more salt and pepper.
16. Serve immediately.

Freestyle SmartPoints Per Serving: 6

(Calories 198 | Total Fats 9.1g | Net Carbs: 22g | Protein 6.6g | Fiber: 4.6g)

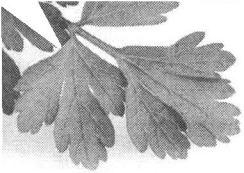

Vegetable Couscous

(Prep Time: 10 MIN | Cook Time: 15 MIN | Serves: 4)

Ingredients:

For cooking:
1 tbsp olive oil

For couscous:
1 cup couscous
1 tomato, chopped
1 cucumber, sliced
1 tbsp lemon juice
¼ cup parsley, chopped

Seasoning:
1 tsp salt
½ tsp dried thyme
¼ tsp black pepper

Directions:

1. Place couscous in the pot and pour in 2 cups of water. Add olive oil, salt, thyme, and pepper.
2. Seal the lid and set the steam release handle to the Sealing position. Press the Manual button and cook for 15 minutes on High pressure.
3. When you hear the cooker's end signal, perform a quick pressure release and open the lid. Cool for a while.
4. Transfer to serving bowl and add vegetables. Sprinkle with lemon juice and some more salt.
5. Serve immediately.

Freestyle SmartPoints Per Serving: 6

(Calories 209 | Total Fats 4g | Net Carbs: 34.2g | Protein 6.3g | Fiber: 2.9g)

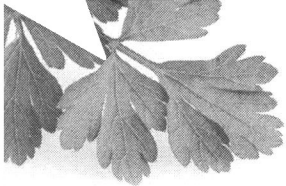

Mini Mushroom Tart

(Prep Time: 15 MIN | Cook Time: 25 MIN | Serves: 4)

Ingredients:

For cooking:

1 tbsp olive oil

For tart:

10oz spinach, chopped
1 onion, chopped
1 lb button mushrooms, sliced
2 oz cottage cheese
4 (6-inch) pie crust

Seasoning:

Salt and pepper to taste

Directions:

1. Plug in the Instant Pot and press the Sauté button. Grease the inner pot with oil and heat up.
2. Add onions and sprinkle with some salt. Cook for 2-3 minutes.
3. Now add mushrooms and continue to cook until all the liquid has evaporated.
4. Finally, add spinach and season with some more salt and pepper. Remove from the pot and transfer to a bowl. Set aside.
5. Pour in 1 cup of water in the inner pot and position a trivet.
6. Place the pie crusts in 4 mini tart pans and add ¼ of the spinach mixture in each. Scatter the cheese on top and loosely cover with aluminum foil.
7. Place tart pans on the trivet and seal the lid. Set the steam release handle to the Sealing position and press the Manual button.
8. Cook for 20 minutes on high pressure.
9. When done, release the pressure by moving the pressure valve to the Venting position.
10. Open the lid and carefully remove the tart pans. Cool to room temperature and serve.

Freestyle SmartPoints Per Serving: 6

(Calories 168 | Total Fats 8.1g | Net Carbs: 15.7g | Protein 8.5g | Fiber: 3.5g)

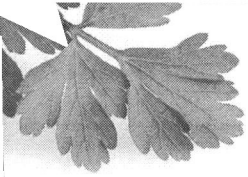

Warm Gazpacho

(Prep Time: 10 MIN | Cook Time: 3-4 MIN | Serves: 2)

Ingredients:

For cooking:
1 tbsp olive oil
½ tsp sherry vinegar
¼ tsp red wine vinegar

For tart:
2 tomatoes, chopped
2 bell peppers, chopped
2 cucumbers, sliced
1 garlic clove, minced
¼ cup cottage cheese

Seasoning:
Salt and pepper to taste

Directions:

1. Place tomatoes in a food processor and puree until smooth.
2. Add the remaining ingredients and process until mostly smooth. Set aside.
3. Plug in the Instant Pot and press the Sauté button. Pour in the tomato mixture and season with salt and pepper.
4. Cook for 3-4 minutes.
5. Press the Cancel button and stir in the cheese.
6. Mix well and serve immediately.

Freestyle SmartPoints Per Serving: 5

(Calories 193 | Total Fats 8.4g | Net Carbs: 21.7g | Protein 8.2g | Fiber: 4.6g)

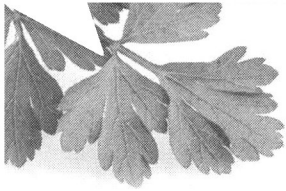

Easy Spinach and Cheese Pizza

(Prep Time: 20 MIN | Cook Time: 25 MIN | Serves: 4)

Ingredients:

For cooking:
1 tbsp olive oil

For pizza:
2 cups spinach, torn
1 cup mozzarella, sliced
3 tbsp tomato paste
1 pizza crust

Seasoning:
¼ tsp garlic powder
¼ tsp dried oregano
½ tsp salt
¼ tsp coconut sugar
¼ tsp white pepper

Directions:

1. Plug in the Instant Pot and press the Sauté button. Add tomato paste, one tablespoon of olive oil, garlic powder, salt, pepper, sugar, and oregano. Pour in about ¼ cup of water and bring it to a boil. Cook for 2-3 minutes, stirring constantly. Press the Cancel button and transfer to a bowl. Set aside.

2. Roll out the pizza crust to fit into round baking pan. Pour the tomato mixture on top and set aside.

3. Press the Sauté button again and heat the remaining olive oil. Add spinach and sprinkle with salt and garlic powder.

4. Cook until wilted and press the Cancel button. Remove from the pot and sprinkle over the pizza crust. Top with mozzarella and loosely cover with aluminum foil. Set aside.

5. Position a trivet at the bottom of the inner pot and pour in 1 cup of water. Place the baking pan on top and seal the lid.

6. Set the steam release handle and press the Manual button. Cook for 15 minutes on High pressure.

7. When done, perform a quick pressure release and open the lid. Remove the pizza from the pot and serve immediately.

Freestyle SmartPoints Per Serving: 3

(Calories 103 | Total Fats 5.4g | Net Carbs: 9.7g | Protein 4.2g | Fiber: 1.1g)

DESSERTS

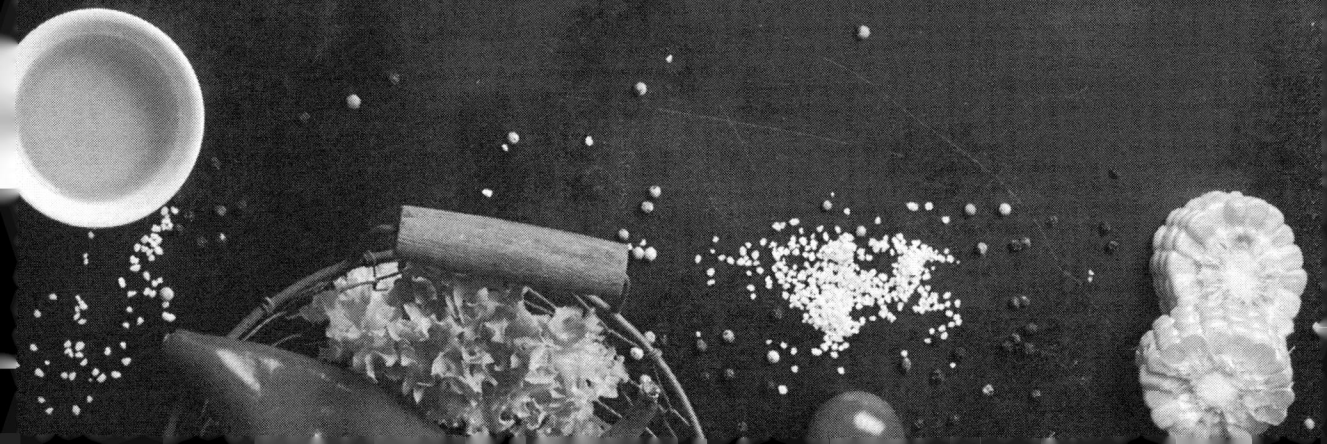

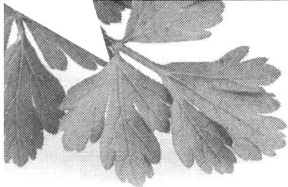

Choc Chip Banana Bread

(Prep Time: 10 MIN | Cook Time: 50 MIN | Serves: 10)

Ingredients:

For cooking:
Nonstick spray

For wet mixture:
⅓ cup brown sugar
1 medium egg
1 tsp vanilla
1½ cups mashed banana
⅓ cup applesauce

For dry mixture:
½ cup cocoa powder
(unsweetened)
1 cup flour
1 tsp bicarb of soda
¼ cup milk choc chips

Directions:

1. Preheat the main oven to 350 degrees F and spritz a loaf tin with nonstick spray.
2. Add all of the wet ingredients to a bowl and whisk to combine.
3. Add the dry ingredients (excluding the choc chips) to a small bowl and stir. Mix the dry ingredients into the wet ingredients until combined and then fold in approximately ¾ of the milk choc chips.
4. Transfer the batter to the loaf tin and scatter with the remaining choc chips. Place in the oven and bake for just under an hour, until set in the center.
5. Allow to cool before removing from the tin and slicing. Serve at room temperature.

Freestyle SmartPoints Per Serving: 4

(Calories 145 | Total Fats 3g | Net Carbs: 25.5g | Protein 3g | Fiber: 3g)

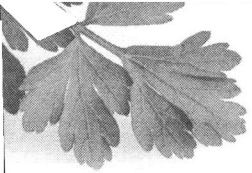

Cookie Crumble Double Choc Muffins

(Prep Time: 10 MIN | Cook Time: 20 MIN | Serves: 12)

Ingredients:

For cooking:
Nonstick spray

For wet mixture:
1 medium egg
2 tbsp liquid egg white
⅓ cup applesauce
(unsweetened)
2 tbsp granulated sugar
1 tsp vanilla essence
¾ cup skim milk

For dry mixture:
1¼ cups flour
⅓ cup cocoa powder
(unsweetened)
1 tsp baking powder
½ tsp bicarb of soda
2 tbsp milk choc chips
4 low-fat cookies 'n crème
sandwich biscuits (crushed)

Directions:

1. Preheat the main oven to 350 degrees F and spritz a 12-hole muffin tin with nonstick spray.
2. Add all of the wet ingredients to a bowl and whisk to combine.
3. Add the dry ingredients (excluding the choc chips and biscuits) to a small bowl and stir. Mix the dry ingredients into the wet ingredients until combined and then fold in the milk choc chips.
4. Transfer the batter to the muffin tin and sprinkle with the crushed biscuits. Place in the oven and bake for 20 minutes.
5. Allow to cool before removing from the tin and serving.

Freestyle SmartPoints Per Serving: 4

(Calories 100 | Total Fats 2.5g | Net Carbs: 15.5g | Protein 3.5g | Fiber: 1.5g)

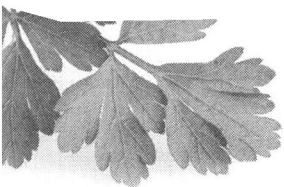

Cookies 'n Crème Swirl Cheesecake Bites

(Prep Time: 2 HOUR 15 MIN | Cook Time: 25 MIN | Serves: 12)

Ingredients:

For cheesecake bites:

12 low-calorie cookies n crème sandwich biscuits

2 tbsp skim milk

½ cup fat-free vanilla Greek yogurt

2½ tbsp granulated sugar

1½ tbsp flour

1 medium egg

1 tbsp low-calorie butter

1 ounces 70% cocoa dark chocolate (melted)

Directions:

1. Preheat the main oven to 325 degrees F and line a 12-hole muffin tin with liners.
2. Place a low-calorie biscuit in the base of each liner.
3. To a bowl, add the remaining cheesecake ingredients (excluding the melted chocolate) and beat until combined.
4. Divide the cheesecake mixture between the liners.
5. Drop a dot of melted chocolate on top of each cheesecake and use a cocktail stick to gently swirl the melted chocolate into the cheesecake.
6. Place in the oven and bake for just under half an hour, until set.
7. Allow to cool before transferring to the refrigerator for a couple of hours and then serving.

Freestyle SmartPoints Per Serving: 4

(Calories 110 | Total Fats 5.5g | Net Carbs: 10.5g | Protein 3.5g | Fiber: 0.5g)

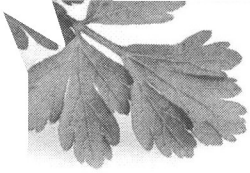

Glazed Donuts

(Prep Time: 40 MIN | Cook Time: 20 MIN | Serves: 6)

Ingredients:

For cooking:
Nonstick spray

For donuts:
⅓ cup low-fat sour cream
2 tbsp granulated sugar
1 medium egg
1 tsp vanilla essence
2½ tbsp fat-free plain yogurt
½ cup + 2 tbsp flour
Pinch kosher salt
1 tsp baking powder

For glaze:
1 tbsp skim milk
2 tbsp powdered sugar

Directions:

1. Preheat the main oven to 325 degrees F and spritz a 6-hole donut tin with nonstick spray.
2. Add all donut ingredients to a mixing bowl and beat until totally combined.
3. Divide the mixture between the holes of the donut tin and place in the oven, bake for just under 20 minutes.
4. Allow to cool completely.
5. Combine the icing ingredients in a shallow bowl and lightly dip the top of each cooled donut into the mixture to coat. Set aside for 10 minutes to set.

Freestyle SmartPoints Per Serving: 4

(Calories 110 | Total Fats 2g | Net Carbs: 18.5g | Protein 9.5g | Fiber: 0.5g)

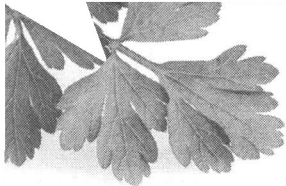

Iced Carrot Cake Loaf with Walnuts

(Prep Time: 30 MIN | Cook Time: 50 MIN | Serves: 10)

Ingredients:

For cooking:
Nonstick spray

For wet mixture:
2 medium eggs

2 tbsp brown sugar

1/3 cup fat-free plain yogurt

1/2 cup applesauce

1 tsp vanilla essence

For dry mixture:
1 tsp cinnamon

1/2 tsp nutmeg

1 1/2 cups flour

1 tsp baking powder

1 tsp bicarb of soda

2 cups carrot (peeled, shredded)

For icing:
1/4 cup low-fat cream cheese

1/4 cup powdered sugar

1/2 tbsp low-calorie butter (at room temperature)

1/2 tsp vanilla essence

1/4 cup walnuts (chopped)

Directions:

1. Preheat the main oven to 375 degrees F and spritz a loaf tin with nonstick spray.
2. Add the wet ingredients to a bowl and beat until combined.
3. In a second bowl, combine all of the dry ingredients (excluding the carrot) and stir. Mix the dry ingredients into the wet ingredients until combined and then fold in the shredded carrot.
4. Transfer the batter to the loaf tin and place in the oven. Bake for just over 45 minutes until set in the center.
5. While the loaf cooks, add all of the icing ingredients (excluding the walnuts) to a bowl and mix with a fork until combined. Keep the icing chilled until ready to use.
6. Remove the loaf from the oven and set aside to cool before spreading the top with the icing and sprinkling with chopped walnuts. Slice and enjoy.

Freestyle SmartPoints Per Serving: 4

(Calories 140 | Total Fats 3g | Net Carbs: 18.5g | Protein 7.5g | Fiber: 0.5g)

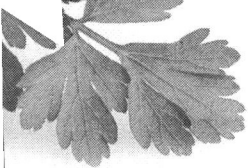

Juicy Peach Dumplings

(Prep Time: 10 MIN | Cook Time: 30 MIN | Serves: 8)

Ingredients:

For peaches:

2 tbsp cornstarch

2 ripe peaches (stoned, peeled, chopped)

2 tbsp brown sugar

For dough:

1 (8 ounce) can low-fat crescent roll dough

2 tbsp cinnamon sugar

Directions:

1. Preheat the main oven to 350 degrees F.
2. Add all of the peach ingredients to a bowl and toss gently until well combined.
3. Separate the dough into the 8 pre-marked triangles.
4. Place equal spoonfuls of peach in the center of each dough triangle and gather the corners of the dough up to surround the filling. Pinch to seal.
5. Arrange the dumplings in a baking dish and sprinkle with cinnamon sugar.
6. Place in the oven and bake for just over half an hour until browned and golden and enjoy while still warm.

Freestyle SmartPoints Per Serving: 5

(Calories 125 | Total Fats 4.5g | Net Carbs: 14g | Protein 2.5g | Fiber: 8g)

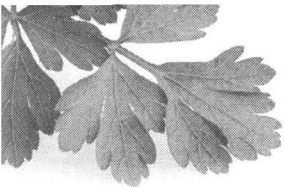

Vanilla and Banana Tapioca Pudding

(Prep Time: 55 MIN | Cook Time: 15 MIN | Serves: 6)

Ingredients:

For pudding:

½ tsp vanilla essence

14 ounces low-fat coconut milk (unsweetened)

¼ cup granulated sugar

4 ripe bananas (peeled, chopped)

1 tbsp + 2 tsp small pearl tapioca (soaked in water for 60 minutes)

Directions:

1. Add the vanilla, coconut milk, and sugar in a saucepan over moderate heat, cook while stirring, until the sugar dissolves.
2. Take off the heat and set aside to cool for several minutes.
3. Return the saucepan of milk to low heat and add the chopped banana and soaked tapioca.
4. Cook for 5 minutes, until the mixture thickens.
5. Take off the heat again and allow to cool completely, before transferring to the refrigerator and chilling until cold.

Freestyle SmartPoints Per Serving: 5

(Calories 165 | Total Fats 6g | Net Carbs: 28g | Protein 2g | Fiber: 2g)

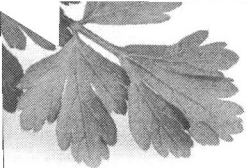

White Chocolate and Raspberry Bread Pudding

(Prep Time: 15 MIN | Cook Time: 20 MIN | Serves: 4)

Ingredients:

For cooking:

Nonstick spray

For pudding:

1 (7½ ounce) can biscuit dough

1 tbsp granulated sugar

1 tsp cinnamon

1 cup fresh raspberries

¼ cup low calories raspberry jam (heated until runny)

1½ tbsp white mini choc chips

Directions:

1. Preheat 350 degrees F, spritz an 8" round dish with nonstick spray and set to one side.
2. Separate the dough into 10 equal pieces and slice each piece into quarters.
3. Add the sugar and cinnamon to a Ziplock bag and shake once to combine, add the dough pieces to the bag and shake again to coat them in the cinnamon sugar.
4. Arrange the coated dough pieces in the dish and scatter with the raspberries. Drizzle over the raspberry jam.
5. Place in the oven and bake for just over 20 minutes. Sprinkle with the white choc chips and set aside for 5-10 minutes until the chips melt a little. Slice and serve warm.

Freestyle SmartPoints Per Serving: 8

(Calories 195 | Total Fats 3.5g | Net Carbs: 38g | Protein 4g | Fiber: 1g)

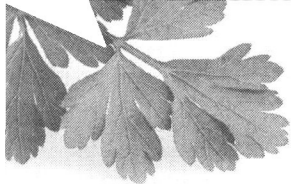

Almond, Chocolate, and Coconut Truffles

(Prep Time: 4 HOUR 10 MIN | Cook Time: N/A | Serves: 28)

Ingredients:

For truffles:

1 ripe, large avocado (peeled, pitted)

¼ cup + 2 tbsp cocoa powder (unsweetened)

½ tsp vanilla essence

1 tsp almond essence

⅔ cup milk choc chips (melted)

For rolling:

½ cup sweetened flaked coconut

Directions:

1. Add the avocado flesh to a food processor and blitz until smooth. Add the remaining truffle ingredients to the processor and blitz until smooth and combined; the mixture should be lump-free.
2. Transfer the truffle mixture to a bowl and cover with plastic wrap, chill for 3-4 hours.
3. Add the flaked coconut to a shallow dish.
4. Using a teaspoon, roll the chilled truffle mixture into 28 smooth balls.
5. Roll each ball in the flaked coconut to coat.
6. Keep chilled until ready to serve.

Freestyle Smart Points Per Serving: 2

(Calories 43 | Total Fats 3g | Net Carbs: 4.5g | Protein 0.5g | Fiber: 0.5g)

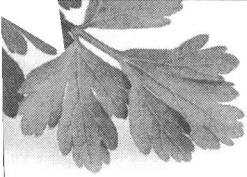

Apple Pie Cookies

(Prep Time: 10 MIN | Cook Time: 12 MIN | Serves: 24)

Ingredients:

For cooking:
Nonstick spray

For cookies:
½ cup applesauce
(unsweetened)
1 (16 ounce) box yellow
sugar-free cake mix
2 medium eggs
½ tsp ground cinnamon
1 cup apples (cored, diced)

Directions:

1. Preheat the main oven to 375 degrees F. Line two cookie sheets with parchment and spritz nonstick spray.
2. Combine the applesauce, cake mix, eggs, and cinnamon in a mixing bowl.
3. Fold in the diced apple until evenly distributed.
4. Use an ice-cream scoop or spoon, to scoop 1" balls of cookie dough onto the prepared sheets. Space the balls of dough a couple of inches apart.
5. Place in the oven and bake for just over 10 minutes.
6. Allow to cool a little before serving.

Freestyle Smart Points Per Serving: 2

(Calories 83 | Total Fats 1.5g | Net Carbs: 16g | Protein 1g | Fiber: 1g)

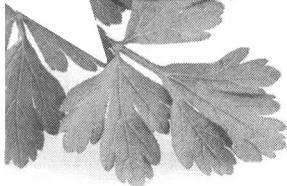

Baked Pears with Cinnamon and Walnuts

(Prep Time: 10 MIN | Cook Time: 30 MIN | Serves: 2)

Ingredients:

For pears:

1 Bartlett pear (halved lengthwise)

1 tsp light brown sugar

Pinch ground cinnamon

1 tbsp walnuts (chopped)

1 (¾ ounce) triangle soft white Cheddar cheese (softened)

Directions:

1. Using a spoon, scoop the core and seeds from the pear halves to form a well.
2. Sprinkle ½ tsp of sugar and a pinch of cinnamon over each pear half.
3. Place ½ tbsp chopped walnuts in the well of each pear half.
4. Place the filled pears in a baking dish (cut-side up). Place in the oven and bake for half an hour.
5. When ready to serve, place the baked pears on plates.
6. Use a spreading knife to 'whip' up the cheese triangle until smooth.
7. Place a spoonful of cheese on top of each pear half and serve hot.

Freestyle Smart Points Per Serving: 2

(Calories 100 | Total Fats 1.5g | Net Carbs: 13g | Protein 1g | Fiber: 3g)

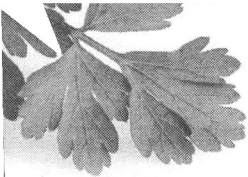

Bite-Sized Pecan Pies

(Prep Time: 10 MIN | Cook Time: 12 MIN | Serves: 15)

Ingredients:

For pecan pies:

15 mini phyllo pastry cups
½ cup pecans (chopped)
¼ cup light brown sugar
2 tbsp half & half
½ tsp vanilla essence
Pinch kosher salt

Directions:

1. Preheat the main oven to 350 degrees F and cover a baking sheet with aluminum foil.
2. Arrange the phyllo pastry cups on the baking sheet.
3. Add the remaining pie ingredients to a bowl and stir to combine. Spoon the filling into the pastry cups.
4. Place in the oven and bake for just over 10 minutes, until golden.
5. Serve warm.

Freestyle Smart Points Per Serving: 2

(Calories 60 | Total Fats 4g | Net Carbs: 6g | Protein 1g | Fiber: 0g)

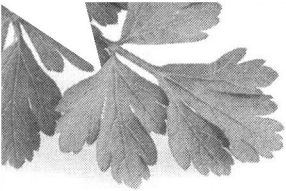

Fruity Pizzas

(Prep Time: 10 MIN | Cook Time: 2 MIN | Serves: 2)

Ingredients:

For ice cream:

2 small low-calorie flatbreads

2 tbsp cream cheese
(whipped)

1 tsp confectioner's sugar

Fruit:

1 large strawberry (hulled,
sliced)

1 large pineapple chunk
(chopped)

4 mandarin segments

2 slices kiwi

6 blueberries

Directions:

1. Toast the flatbreads until lightly golden.

2. Combine the whipped cream cheese and confectioner's sugar in a small bowl.

3. Spread each flatbread with an equal amount of the cream cheese mixture.

4. Divide the fruit between the two 'pizzas' and enjoy.

Freestyle Smart Points Per Serving: 3

(Calories 110 | Total Fats 3g | Net Carbs: 17g | Protein 4g | Fiber: 2g)

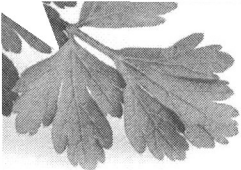

Guilt-Free Brownies

(Prep Time: 10 MIN | Cook Time: 35 MIN | Serves: 12)

Ingredients:

For cooking:
Nonstick spray

For wet mixture:
1½ cups canned black beans
(drained, rinsed)
¼ cup blackstrap molasses
¼ cup applesauce
(unsweetened)

For dry mixture:
⅓ cup cocoa powder
(unsweetened)
¼ cup all-purpose flour
½ tsp kosher salt
½ tsp baking powder

Directions:

1. Preheat the main oven to 375 degrees F. Spritz an 8" square baking dish with nonstick spray.
2. Add the black beans to a blender, blitz until smooth and chunk-free. Transfer the black beans to a bowl along with the blackstrap molasses and applesauce. Mix well.
3. Add all of the dry ingredients to the black bean mixture and stir well until totally combined.
4. Transfer the brownie batter to the baking dish and place in the oven. Bake for just over half an hour.
5. Allow to cool to room temperature before slicing and serving.

Freestyle Smart Points Per Serving: 1

(Calories 120 | Total Fats 1g | Net Carbs: 19g | Protein 6g | Fiber: 5g)

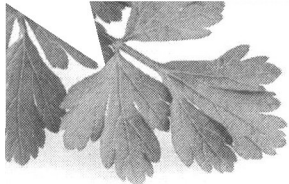

Key Lime Pie Bites

(Prep Time: 10 MIN | Cook Time: 17 MIN | Serves: 12)

Ingredients:

For key lime bites:

12 low-fat vanilla wafers

8 ounces low-fat cream cheese
(at room temperature)

1 (5¼ ounce) container fat-free
Key lime flavor Greek yogurt

⅓ cup granulated sugar

1 egg (beaten)

1 tbsp freshly squeezed lime
juice

For topping:

12 tbsp low-fat whip cream

Directions:

1. Preheat the main oven to 375 degrees F. Fill a 12-hole cupcake tin with liners.

2. Place a vanilla wafer in the base of each liner.

3. Add the remaining key lime ingredients to a bowl and combine using an electric whisk until fluffy and smooth. Spoon an equal amount of the mixture into each liner on top of the wafer.

4. Place in the oven and bake for just over 15 minutes. Set aside to cool completely before transferring to the refrigerator for an hour.

5. Top each bite with 1 tbsp whip cream.

Freestyle Smart Points Per Serving: 4

(Calories 105 | Total Fats 6g | Net Carbs: 10g | Protein 3g | Fiber: 0g)

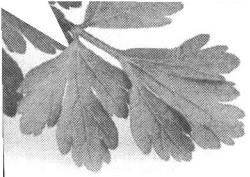

Mini Lemon and Strawberry Cheesecakes

(Prep Time: 3 HOUR 10 MIN | Cook Time: 5 MIN | Serves: 30)

Ingredients:

For cheesecakes:

30 mini phyllo pastry cups

8 ounces low-fat cream cheese (softened)

¼ cup fat-free Greek yogurt

2 tbsp granulated sugar

2 tsp freshly squeezed lemon juice

1 tsp lemon zest (finely grated)

1 tsp vanilla essence

For topping:

5 large strawberries (hulled, sliced into 6 pieces each)

5 slices lemon (sliced into 6 mall triangles each)

Directions:

1. Preheat the main oven to 350 degrees F.
2. Arrange the phyllo cups on a baking sheet and place in the oven for 5 minutes until golden. Set aside to cool.
3. Add the remaining cheesecake ingredients to a mixing bowl and whisk until fluffy and combined. Transfer the mixture to a piping bag.
4. Pipe the cheesecake mixture into the cooled phyllo cups and garnish each with a small piece of strawberry and lemon.
5. Chill the cheesecakes for 3 hours before serving.

Freestyle Smart Points Per Serving: 2

(Calories 70 | Total Fats 2.5g | Net Carbs: 9.5g | Protein 2g | Fiber: 0g)

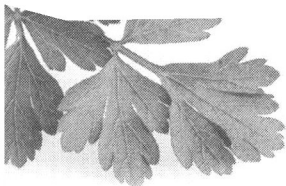

Peanut Butter Cookie Dough Balls

(Prep Time: 3 HOUR 10 MIN | Cook Time: N/A | Serves: 36)

Ingredients:

For cookie dough balls:

¾ cup canned chickpeas
(drained, rinsed)

3 tbsp organic smooth peanut
butter

⅓ cup brown sugar

1 tsp low-fat cream cheese

½ tsp vanilla essence

¼ tsp kosher salt

⅛ tsp bicarb of soda

2 tbsp all-purpose flour

2 tbsp peanut butter chips

For rolling:

2 tbsp cocoa powder
(unsweetened)

2 tbsp confectioner's sugar

Directions:

1. Add all cookie dough ball ingredients (excluding the peanut butter chips) to a food processor and blitz until smooth and combined.

2. Add the peanut butter chips and pulse until incorporated. Transfer the cookie dough to a bowl, cover with plastic wrap and chill for an hour.

3. Combine the cocoa powder and confectioner's sugar in a shallow bowl.

4. Roll the chilled cookie dough into 36 equal balls, and roll each ball in the cocoa/sugar mixture.

5. Keep chilled until ready to serve.

Freestyle Smart Points Per Serving: 1

(Calories 32 | Total Fats 1g | Net Carbs: 4.5g | Protein 1g | Fiber: 1g)

INSTANT POT DESSERTS

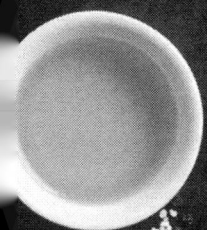

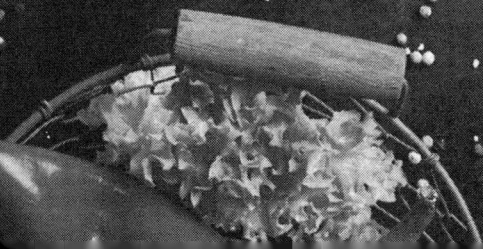

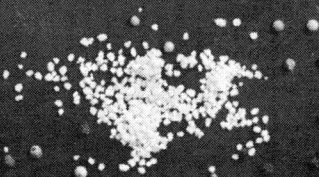

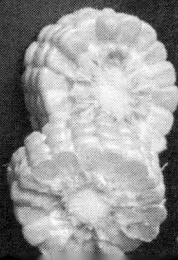

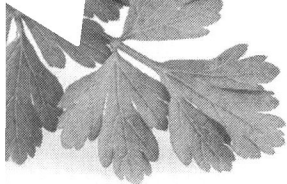

Rum Bundt Cake

(Prep Time: 15 MIN | Cook Time: 40 MIN | Serves: 10)

Ingredients:

For cooking:

Nonstick cooking spray

For cake:

1 cup all-purpose flour

1 tbsp butter, unsalted

¾ cup Swerve

1 large egg

2 large egg whites

5 oz cream cheese, low-fat

½ tsp baking powder

¼ tsp salt

1 tsp rum extract

Directions:

1. Grease a fitting Bundt pan with some nonstick cooking spray and set aside.
2. In a large mixing bowl, combine flour, baking powder, swerve, and salt. Stir until combined and set aside.
3. In a separate large mixing bowl, combine butter, egg, egg whites, cream cheese, and rum extract. Beat with a hand mixer until well incorporated.
4. Now, pour the wet ingredients over dry ingredients and mix until combined.
5. Pour the mixture into the prepared Bundt pan and set aside.
6. Plug in the Instant Pot and pour 1 cup of water in the stainless steel insert. Set the trivet on the bottom of the pot and place the pan on top. Cover the pan with some aluminum foil and close the lid. Adjust the steam release handle and press the Manual button. Set the timer for 40 minutes and cook on High pressure.
7. When done, perform a quick pressure release and open the lid. Transfer the pan to a wire rack and let it chill for a while.
8. Optionally, serve with some Mascarpone cheese and enjoy!

Freestyle SmartPoints Per Serving: 4

(Calories 117 | Total Fats 6.7g | Net Carbs: 9.7g | Protein 3.7g | Fiber: 0.4g)

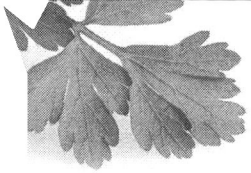

Lime Pudding

(Prep Time: 15 MIN | Cook Time: 40 MIN | Serves: 6)

Ingredients:

For cooking:

Nonstick cooking spray

2 cups water

For pudding:

2 oz vanilla pudding mix, sugar-free

1 envelope gelatin, sugar-free

1 tsp lime extract

½ cup Cool Whip, fat-free

Directions:

1. Plug in your Instant Pot and pour in the water.
2. Press the Sauté button and add pudding mix. Bring it to a boil and stir constantly.
3. Now, add gelatin mix and lime extract. Cook for 2 more minutes, stirring constantly.
4. Pour the mixture into serving bowls or ramekins. Let it cool completely.
5. Top each bowl with Cool Whip and refrigerate for 15 minutes before serving.
6. Enjoy!

Freestyle SmartPoints Per Serving: 2

(Calories 49 | Total Fats 1.6g | Net Carbs: 7.4g | Protein 1.1g | Fiber: 0g)

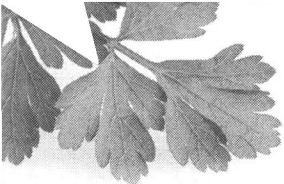

Cinnamon Peach Bake

(Prep Time: 15 MIN | Cook Time: 2 HOURS | Serves: 4)

Ingredients:

For cooking:

Nonstick cooking spray

For peaches:

4 large peaches, sliced

3 tbsp raisins

4 tbsp granulated Stevia

1 tsp cinnamon powder

1 tsp butter

Directions:

1. Wash the peaches and cut into halves. Remove the pits and cut each half into 3 slices. Set aside.

2. Plug in the Instant Pot and grease the stainless steel insert with some nonstick cooking spray.

3. Place the peach slices and raisins in the inner pot. Sprinkle with cinnamon powder and granulated stevia. Spoon the butter on top and securely lock the lid. Adjust the steam release handle by moving the valve to the Sealing position. Set the Slow Cooker mode and cook for 2 hours on Low pressure.

4. When done, release the pressure naturally. Open the lid and transfer all to a serving dish.

5. Chill for a while before serving.

Freestyle SmartPoints Per Serving: 2

(Calories 88 | Total Fats 1.4g | Net Carbs: 16.8g | Protein 1.6g | Fiber: 2.6g)

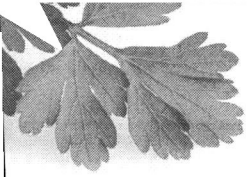

Chocolate Mini Fudge Cakes

(Prep Time: 20 MIN | Cook Time: 30 MIN | Serves: 8)

Ingredients:

For mini fudge cakes:

5 oz unsweetened dark chocolate, roughly chopped

½ cup sugar

6 large marshmallows

2 tsp margarine, reduced-calorie

2 tbsp evaporated milk

Directions:

1. Plug in the Instant Pot and press the Sauté button. Add margarine and milk. Gently stir until the margarine has been completely melted.

2. Stir in the sugar and bring it all to a boil. Cook for 1 minute, stirring constantly.

3. Add chocolate and stir until all well combined and creamy.

4. Turn off the pot and add marshmallows. Stir again until melted. Transfer the mixture into small ramekins and set aside to cool completely.

5. Refrigerate for 1 hour before serving.

6. Enjoy!

Freestyle SmartPoints Per Serving: 7

(Calories 138 | Total Fats 6.2g | Net Carbs: 25.5g | Protein 0.7g | Fiber: 1.1g)

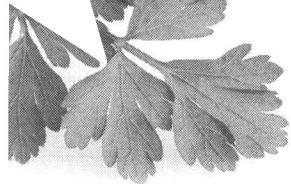

Blueberry Mug Cake

(Prep Time: 5 MIN | Cook Time: 20 MIN | Serves: 2)

Ingredients:

For cooking:

Nonstick cooking spray

For mug cake:

½ cup blueberries

1 large egg

3 tbsp all-purpose flour

2 tbsp cocoa powder, raw

2 tsp powdered stevia

¼ tsp baking powder

¼ tsp blueberry extract

¼ tsp salt

Directions:

1. Combine all-purpose flour, cocoa powder, stevia, and baking powder in a mixing bowl. Mix until combined and then add the remaining ingredients. Beat well until a fine batter has been formed.

2. Grease an oven-safe mug or ramekin with some nonstick cooking spray. Fill about 2/3 of the mug. Optionally, top with some dark chocolate chips.

3. Plug in the Instant Pot and pour 1 cup of water in the stainless steel insert. Set the trivet and place the mug on top. Close the lid and adjust the steam release handle by moving the valve to the Sealing position. Cook on Manual mode for 20 minutes over High pressure.

4. When done, perform a quick pressure release by moving the valve to the Venting position. Open the lid and transfer the mug to a wire rack. Let it cool completely before serving.

Freestyle SmartPoints Per Serving: 3

(Calories 112 | Total Fats 3.4g | Net Carbs: 14.8g | Protein 5.6g | Fiber: 2.8g)

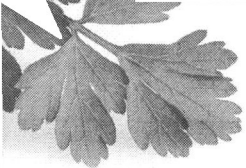

New York Style Cheesecake

(Prep Time: 20 MIN | Cook Time: 25 MIN | Serves: 10)

Ingredients:

For cooking:

1 tbsp butter, melted

For cheesecake:

3 large eggs

1 lbs cream cheese

1 cups Greek yogurt, fat-free

¼ cup whipped cream, fat-free

1 tsp vanilla extract

1 cup Swerve

½ tsp salt

½ tsp ginger powder

Directions:

1. Grease the bottom of a spring-form pan with butter and tightly wrap the pan with aluminum foil. Set aside.
2. In a large mixing bowl, beat eggs and swerve until light and fluffy. Add cream cheese and continue to beat until creamy texture.
3. Pour in the Greek yogurt and whipped cream. Sprinkle with vanilla extract, salt, and ginger powder.
4. Continue to beat for 3-4 minutes on high speed.
5. Pour the mixture into the pan and loosely cover with some more aluminum foil.
6. Plug in the Instant Pot and position a trivet at the bottom of the inner pot. Pour in 2 cups of water and place the wrapped spring-form pan in it.
7. Seal the lid and set the steam release handle to the Sealing position. Cook for 25 minutes on high pressure.
8. When done, perform a quick pressure release and open the lid.
9. Remove the pan from the pot and cool to room temperature. Refrigerate overnight before serving.

Freestyle SmartPoints Per Serving: 8

(Calories 201 | Total Fats 18.2g | Net Carbs: 2.3g | Protein 7.6g | Fiber: 0g)

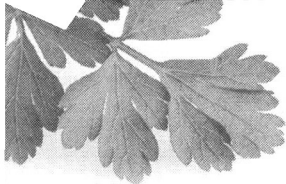

Conclusion

Well Freestyle chefs, that's it! You now have everything you need to embark on your new Freestyle journey towards a healthier, happier you. From breakfast to lunch, snack time to dinner, desserts to soup, and everything in between, you can now enjoy all of your favorite dishes without the unnecessary fats, sugars, or general "yuck." The sky is truly the limit when it comes to the meals you can prepare with the new Freestyle diet, and we bet your kitchen will become the next go-to healthy hot spot in the neighbourhood in no time at all!

The only thing left to do is dig into the back of your closet, dust off those skinny jeans, and get ready to strut your stuff because you'll be fitting back into them before you know it!

Made in the USA
Lexington, KY
27 June 2018